Intermittent Fasting For Women Over 50:

The Complete Beginner's Guide to Lose Weight, Promote Longevity, Increase Energy, and Support Hormones. Detox and Rejuvenate your Body with a Healthy Lifestyle

AMY STEPHENS

Table of Contents

Introduction

You are likely already familiar with the term 'fasting,' perhaps having heard it about religious practices or something you had to do before blood tests or an operation. It most likely creates an image in your head of draconian practices in which people punish themselves for their sins. You may think that fasting means not eating. Intermittent fasting, however, has nothing to do with starving yourself. The term 'starvation' implies that you do not have access to food and that you are, in some way, experiencing negative health effects from not eating. Starvation is generally not deliberate or controlled.

Instead, intermittent fasting means that although you do have access to food, you *choose* when to eat and the experience is not damaging to your health in the way that starvation would be. Intermittent fasting involves assigning a pattern for eating around specific times.

You may be wondering how that is any different from eating breakfast, lunch, and dinner at specific times. If you consider the fact that you usually don't eat meals at specific times but rather when and if you are hungry, that shows a distinct difference between the two ideas. When you practice intermittent fasting, you structure your day in fasting hours and eating hours. There are various time-based protocols that we will discuss later in this book to attribute different periods to fasting and eating. The essential idea is that you allocate a period of the day in which you do not eat and then a period of the day in which you do eat. Intermittent fasting is different from other eating plans in that it does not determine what you can eat but rather when you should eat.

The term "intermittent fasting" was the most popular diet-related reference in search engines in 2019 with a 10,000 percent increase in the search for this term since 2010 (Fung, 2020). One of the most popular intermittent fasting methods that we can use to illustrate the concept is the 16:8 protocol. In this protocol, you fast for 16 hours and then you have an eating window of eight hours. Considering you are already not eating while you sleep, which should ideally be for eight hours, the idea is to extend that period for another eight hours. Therefore, this would mean if you go to sleep at 10 pm and wake up at 6 am, you would then not eat until 2 pm. From 2 pm to 10 pm, you can eat a small light lunch and then dinner at least two hours before you go to sleep for digestion purposes.

This is the basis of intermittent fasting, which, in itself, will provide you with a myriad of health benefits. If you decide that you also want to lose a certain amount of weight specifically, you will need to limit the number of calories you take in during your eating window and increase your activity. You should take in no food during your fasting window, but you can drink beverages that have little to no caloric content such as water or coffee and tea with no milk or sugar. You can take supplements during your fasting period. Still, if possible, you may want to delay taking the supplements until your eating period since taking them on an empty stomach can make you feel nauseous.

Intermittent fasting is a very natural way of structuring our eating. Before we had a constant supply of food on demand, fasting was the norm, and it is still a very natural process for many animals, some of which don't eat for weeks or months at a time while hibernating. After all, our hunter-gatherer ancestors did not have the luxury of constant access to food, so fasting was not a choice for them, but they survived some challenging conditions all the same.

Of course, our energy requirements are very different today than during the age that we had to hunt our food. At that time, we needed bursts of energy to overcome situations that occasionally cropped up. Today, our energy requirements are more sustained, so it stands to reason that we would not fast for extended periods.

It does take a mindset change to introduce intermittent fasting as a lifestyle since you have likely grown up with the idea that having three square meals per day is the healthiest way to eat. We have also had phrases like "breakfast is the most important meal of the day" drummed into our heads, usually just a marketing tool for sugar-filled cereal brands.

An intermittent fasting lifestyle has many health benefits including weight loss, fat burning, stabilization of blood sugar, limiting of disease, increased rate of cell repair, and increased longevity.

In explaining what intermittent fasting is, it is perhaps pertinent to explain what it is not. Intermittent fasting is not a free ticket to binge on everything your eyes see as long as you 'starve' yourself within the required period. Anyone approaching intermittent fasting from such a standpoint is doing themselves more harm than good. The basics of good nutrition—lean proteins, plenty of fresh fruit and vegetables, good sources of fiber, and good fats—do not change because you are structuring the times you eat. If you wish to see all of the benefits that intermittent fasting can offer, maintaining good nutrition with the occasional treat is imperative.

One of the downsides of the sudden burst in popularity of intermittent fasting is that people will tout it as a fad diet and make recommendations around suggested protocols that are not good for your health. Educating yourself around the principles of fasting as a practice and how your body works when fasting is the key to not being taken in by one of these misguided trends. True intermittent fasting does not describe a condition under which you can continuously overindulge during your eating windows as long as you 'deprive' yourself during your fasting window.

Another essential factor to consider in understanding intermittent fasting is the period for which you fast. Abstaining from food in the intermittent fasting lifestyle is never intended to be prolonged. Some protocols dictate a 24-hour fast fast, and for expert-level fasters, this is fine, but it is not recommended for beginners. Any period longer than 24-hours is not recommended for anyone.

As we will delve into in more in-depth detail later, intermittent fasting is quite flexible as long as you stick to the basic ideas behind it and ensure that you are promoting health. If your goal is weight loss, it is essential to understand that intermittent fasting will help you lose weight relatively quickly, but it does so in a healthy manner. If you do not continue with an intermittent fasting lifestyle after losing the weight you want to, you are at risk of gaining weight again. At the very least, you must commit to maintaining a lower caloric intake and a higher caloric burning through increased activity.

This book gives you a considerable amount of information on intermittent fasting, but it is essential to refresh and recharge your knowledge continuously. Do ensure that you choose your sources of knowledge wisely, though, and stick to reputable experts and websites. The great thing about intermittent fasting is that you will quickly become knowledgeable on the subject just by practicing the lifestyle. As you continue on your journey, if you notice certain things happening in your body that didn't before, do some research to see what processes within the body are causing it. This is how we get to know our bodies. Even at 50, we can learn about our bodies, and it is vital to be open to new possibilities.

Chapter 1 What Is Intermittent Fasting?

Intermittent fasting is nothing but fasting for extended periods and eating only within an allowed window of time. So, what does fasting do and how does it help you lose weight?

Feeding and Fasting

Our body is continuously in one of two states, which are the feeding or fasting states. When we eat a meal, our body is in the feeding state and it remains in this state for the next 4 to 5 hours. We do not feel hungry in this state. After about 6 to 8 hours comes the post feeding state or the intermediate state, where we may or may not feel hungry. The body uses our most recent meal to gather energy when needed for some action. After this comes the fasting stage, which lasts until we have another meal.

We haven't taken a meal during this fasting stage, and our body has already used the last meal to derive energy. It now turns to our stored energy reserves, which are the fats in our body. This is the stage when fats get burned. In this stage we feel hungry and our body looks for food to use as fuel, but upon not finding any recent meal, because we haven't eaten, burns our fat stores. This is why fasting has been known to be such a meaningful way to burn accumulated fats. But if we have provided our body with food, it doesn't enter the fasting stage and no fat gets burned and our body resorts to our next meal for energy.

The Science behind Intermittent Fasting

To understand how intermittent fasting works, it is essential to understand what usually happens in our bodies with the food we eat. Whenever we take a meal, eat or even drink something, our body releases a hormone called insulin. Insulin is widely popular as a medicine given to people with diabetes. Still, not much thought is given to it as to the why and the how of it.

This insulin released at the time of food consumption acts as the monitor of our blood glucose levels. Insulin takes care of the amount of glucose we need immediately as energy for our actions. It decides how much of this glucose should be converted to glycogen, which is nothing but a readily available energy source, and how much of it should be stored as fat for later use. This is the reason why insulin is also known as a fat-storing hormone. Some people with diabetes cannot have this glucose monitor in their blood and hence need external insulin injections to handle their blood glucose levels.

If you are frequently or regularly eating, then your body is regularly releasing insulin. This leads to more and more storage of energy in the form of fats. Your body has no chance to reach your already present fat reserves to burn them for energy; instead, it continually adds to them. One important thing to keep in mind is keeping your insulin levels in check, which can be easily done by adequately scheduling your meals.

Ghrelin is known as the hunger hormone as this is the hormone responsible for causing us hunger and pushing us to eat more. Suppose your regular eating schedule involves three meals a day. In that case, your body secretes the ghrelin hormone at your three mealtimes to signal it is time to eat. Ghrelin release does not necessarily mean your body needs food, it merely means it is your regular eating time and your body reminds you to eat. You can regulate ghrelin levels by intermittent fasting so that your body gets adjusted to your new eating schedules.

Leptin is another important hormone that helps regulate your food intake. It is also called the satiety hormone, because it signals that you have had enough food and hints you to stop eating. It helps you feel full and satisfied. The higher the leptin levels the less likely you are to eat food. Naturally, since birth, we are wired to have a balance of both ghrelin and leptin levels. With our ever-changing lifestyles and unhealthy food practices, that causes this inherent balance to be disturbed. These hormone levels swing either way, causing us to put on more weight through unregulated eating habits.

You see the best demonstration of the working of these hormones in infants and toddlers to some extent. Children in these age groups have their minds of when they would like to eat and how much. This is their hormones talking and they are often doing a better job than us to keep our food intake in check. We often see parents struggling to feed their toddlers, running around the house or the backyard trying to get a few bites in. The thing is, a toddler generally doesn't eat when they are full. Their leptin tells them they have had enough, and they refuse to eat more. We, as concerned parents, sometimes force them to eat. Here begins the imbalance of these hormones. Leptin no longer functions appropriately, because we seem to eat even when it signals us not to. Right from that age, we begin to tell our brains we eat at certain times, or because we have food on hand, or we have something before us that we absolutely cannot pass up. This messes up with the hormone signals. We are not eating like we used to in the infant to toddler age, when we are hungry; instead we eat because it is our supposed mealtime, even if we do not feel the need. All the three hormones, insulin, ghrelin, and leptin, are now in quite an imbalanced state, leading us to feel hungry all the time, causing us to eat all the time, thereby increasing our fat storage.

Six Meals A Day - The Wrong Approach

In most diets, the most popular phenomenon is to divide your whole food intake per day into six or more small portions. These meals are taken throughout the day with a gap of a few hours in between. It has been a popular belief for quite some time now that doing so helps your metabolism and helps reduce weight because you aren't feeding on large quantities at once. Instead, what this truly does is keeps your insulin levels always high. What this does in turn is convert all the digested sugars into fats.

Naturally in a single day, you wouldn't require all the energy that even six small meals could give you. So, the sugar monitor in your blood, insulin, directs all the unused sugars to be turned into fat and stored for later. Doing this day in and day out, every day, simply increases your fat stores. We need to use up the already stored fat not add more to it. But that is precisely what eating several small meals in a day does. Only when we give our body time to reduce its insulin levels in the blood will it be able to access the stored fat and use that for energy. This is impossible when a constant food intake is going on. The time intervals between these small meals are too short to induce our bodies to access the stored fat, because it still has glucose from the most recent meal to make use of.

Therefore, contrary to popular belief, six or more small meals are the wrong way to go about it. The need of the hour is to look for something that gives your body sufficient time to reach those stored fats and burn them, and intermittent fasting is ideal for just that!

Drawbacks of Intermittent Fasting for Women Over 50

Intermittent fasting has a few drawbacks, especially in the beginning stages, when a person is still getting accustomed to retimed eating schedules. These drawbacks are few. For women, who can and cannot apply intermittent fasting schedules, we should decide based on their medical and physical conditions, which we shall look at later on in the book. But once a woman has decided and begun fasting, it is only a matter of adjusting and adapting oneself to the new eating patterns. Whatever disadvantages or drawbacks arise due to intermittent fasting, all stem from this adjustment stage.

Severe hunger pangs, lightheadedness, dizziness, dehydration, headaches, and muscle weakness are problems that people usually face due to intermittent fasting schedules. These are also restricted to the adapting or adjusting stage. One rare drawback of the fasting system is infertility. But this is hardly an issue after a couple of weeks of stopping the schedule and less so for women over 50 who are mostly beyond the child-bearing age.

Chapter 2 How Intermittent Fasting Work

Your body can handle extended periods of not eating. Human bodies have the natural ability to transition between the hunger state and the full state. When we don't eat for a long period, the processes going inside our body change. When we eat our body starts to digest and store the energy received through the meal. When we are hungry, our body starts to take energy from those stored fats.

When we are fasted for a specific period, our blood sugar and insulin levels face a reduction. It is normal because it pushes our body to thrive from existing resources present inside our bodies. Researches have shown that fasting helps protect against diseases like heart diseases, diabetes, cancer and Alzheimer's disease. Therefore, when in a fasted state, you shouldn't worry that you shouldn't worry that it will affect your health.

To understand how intermittent fasting works, two states have to be understood first. The two states are – the fed state and the fasted state. We know how our bodies keep functioning well even though our stomachs are empty or full by understanding these states.

Two IF states: Fed Vs. Fasted

In the Fed state, the body is undergoing process of digesting and absorbing food. The state begins when you start eating and can last from three to five hours after that. In fed state, your body shows elevated insulin levels, which acts as a signal for your body to store excess calories. This storage takes place in the fat cells. During the time with high insulin levels, the process of fat burning comes to a stop and the body shifts towards burning glucose from your last meal instead.

A state called post-absorptive state comes, which lasts about 8 to 12 hours after the last meal. After that the body enters the Fasted state. In the Fasted state; body is not processing any meal and the levels of insulin are low. This induces a mobilization of stored body fat presiding inside the body in the fat cells, and starts to burn these fats for providing energy to the body. In this state, the body can burn the fat that was first inaccessible to it during the fed state.

Staying hungry for a specific duration of time helps you with hundreds of things. When you eat a meal, your body is under 'fed state' and is just processing the meal you just ate. After a few hours pass and the food is completely digested, it goes into a mid-stage where you don't feel hungry but haven't eaten anything else yet. You can call this an intermediate state. After 8 to 12 hours from your last meal, a state comes called 'fasted state' when you feel hungry and you are under a fast. In this state, your body needs to regain the fuel to work but it doesn't find any energy being provided to it. So, it starts to look for energy sources inside the body. The body is designed to store some amount of fat from every meal to regain energy at the time when it is needed. Thus, the body has entered into a fat-burning state because of low insulin levels and starts to burn the fats present inside the body. This is beneficial in hundreds of ways. It will eliminate the excess fat from you and get rid of any toxins present inside a body.

The toxins can be anything harmful present in your body. It can be dysfunctional cell or a cell that is damaged and is not performing well. Removal of such cells is essential when we talk about maintaining health. So, you have to be under the 'fasted state' so that your body can initialize the burn-off state. Intermittent fasting provides you a convenient way to enter into the fasted state and get rid of all excess fats, calories and damaged cells. Many health-practitioners and doctors advise their patients to start fasting for this purpose. They believe that health will improve if they fast because of this quality of intermittent fasting.

How Intermittent Fasting Affects Women at This Age & How to Approach It

Because health, diet, reproductivity, and nutritional needs are all altered for mature and menopausal women, their intermittent fasting relationships can be very different from young women's. For instance, while young women ought to be careful about how intermittent fasting can affect their fertility levels, older women can practice intermittent fasting freely without these concerns. Therefore, more mature women can apply the weight-loss techniques of intermittent fasting to their lives (and waistlines) without worrying about what adverse side effects might arise in the future.

However, for menopausal women, the situation is slightly different from that of fully mature women. People going through menopause have to deal with daily hormone fluctuations that cause hot and cold flashes, sleeplessness, anxiety, irregular periods, and more. At the beginning of this process, intermittent fasting will not necessarily help, and it could even make your situation more stressful.

For women in this situation who are actively going through menopause, you must remember that your body is susceptible to changes right now. Suppose you do find that intermittent fasting helps and that short periods of fast are useful. In that case, you must also make sure to increase your fast intensity as gradually as possible so your body can adjust without creating horrible hormonal repercussions for yourself and everyone around you. For the fully mature woman, intermittent fasting will not make you as cranky, moody, irregular in the period, or otherwise because those hormones won't be affecting you at all anymore, or at least, hardly at all. Your dietary and eating schedule choices become more liberated from the effects they used to have on your hormonal health as the years go by. Therefore, if you're seeking weight loss, better energy, a physiological jolt back to health, or what have you, try out IF without concern and see what happens. For these women, intermittent fasting is set to provide hope through eased depression, the lessened likelihood of cancer (or its recurrence), promised weight loss, and more.

Chapter 3 Myths around Intermittent Fasting

Now that we have seen some intermittent fasting types and chosen which method suits us the most, the next step would be to rid our minds of certain myths that people have initiated about intermittent fasting over the years. One credible characteristic of the human mouth and hands is their ability to talk and write critically. People would always have a different view and not flow in synergy with what is brought to the table irrespective of how prospect-filled it may appear. Certain myths have come up over the years about the concept of intermittent fasting and it would only be to have me address this in this book. Here are a few;

- **Intermittent fasting is a road to starvation**: A little enlightenment on this would be in order. Starvation is a condition where someone suffers severely due to a lack of food. It is wrong to think that not eating for 24-48 hours starves the body. Research has inadvertently shown that for the body to get started and experience a reduction in metabolic rate, an individual has to not eat for over 60 hours. That is almost three days. As individuals, tight work schedules prevent us from eating for a more significant part of the day and even though we expend a lot of energy doing our work, we still do not break down.

- **The burden of hunger**: Some others say that you will feel hungry all day long while doing intermittent fasting. The human body is very adaptive. That is why impoverished or poor individuals can stay for almost a day without food. They are healthy and working tirelessly. From the second week of intermittent fasting, hunger gets low; your body adjusts to your new routine. Just as your body adjusts when saddled with more energy-consuming activities. Here's another thing; most times we are most likely to feel hungry easily when we are in an idle state (doing nothing). Something else you could do is to keep yourself busy all the while during your fasting periods. Getting busy takes our minds away from a lot of things including food, we're fully focused on what we have at hand.

- **Eating frequently boosts your metabolism**: Now it is another myth generally acknowledged by many people that eating often boosts metabolism. We cannot deny that calories are expended in metabolic processes; this is very true. This is also seen in the digestion of food and known as the Thermic Effect of Food. The body uses about 10% of your overall calorie intake to do this. On the other hand, now, here's where this myth is faulting. What matters is not how frequently you eat, but the number of calories you eat. Now someone consuming six diets of about 500 calories is the same as consuming three diets containing a thousand calories. Therefore, this is the wrong myth.

- **Dietary glucose for the brain**: Here's another common misconception. Some people believe that if you do not eat carbs every once in a while, your brain will cease to function. The reason for this is that the brain uses glucose as its only source of fuel. On the other hand, this myth is faulted too because of the concept of gluconeogenesis. This is a process whereby the body synthesizes glucose from non-carbohydrate sources. During long fasts, such as this and low carb dieting, your body can produce ketone bodies from dietary fats. These ketone bodies feed a part of the brain until it significantly reduces its glucose requirements.

Reduction in muscle mass: People have also concluded that intermittent fasting reduces body mass. Although this sometimes happens during fasting, any experiment hasn't proved that it happens more with intermittent fasting than other fast forms. Recent studies show a significant increase in muscle mass for individuals who consume all the calorie requirement in one big meal in a day. It is a predominant technique among bodybuilders, it maintains the muscles. It enhances a considerable amount of weight loss with minimal reduction in muscle mass. This myth is flawed as many evidence proves that intermittent fasts have minimal effect on muscle mass.

- **Incessant eating ensures good health**: People think that when they eat incessantly, they make good health.

This is not entirely true. The body indeed requires nutrients and energy to thrive. Still, Cellular repair processes are engaged during intermittent fast periods. This Cellular repair process known as Autophagy uses dysfunctional and waste proteins for energy. It also prevents aging, cancer and Alzheimer's disease. Some studies have shown that snacking and eating regularly most times harm your body in different ways. For example, when you take a diet with many calories, you cause your liver to become fatty, making you more likely to get fatty liver disease.

Additionally, some research has come up to say that you put yourself more in the danger of colorectal cancer if you eat often. Therefore, this further proves that intermittent fast has more health and metabolic benefits than you could imagine.

- **Skipping breakfast can make you fat**: I also don't know how this myth came about or how it came to be believed. Well, that is how myths are. It is thought that skipping breakfasts increases your meal cravings, thus making you consume more food. However, research has proven that skipping breakfast does not have any signs of individuals' weight gain or otherwise. Therefore, you must pay attention to your specific needs. Breakfast is a must for some people and some others can do without it.

- **Indiscipline eating habits on work days**: Now you engaging in intermittent fasting does not give you the leverage to be glut tonic and eat whatever comes to the eyes. In as much as intermittent fasting helps burn up a lot of calories, replacing the burnt up Calories with even more significant amounts on Fast off days counters productive results. It's like shooting yourself on the leg. You take away a piece of dirt and bring in a basket full. At all times, a healthy eating habits should be maintained. Adequate and healthy calorie consumption should be checked and monitored. This is why it is mostly advised that you begin intermittent fasts with a dietician/doctor's assistance. Do not pull down your longhouse of cards with your own hands; self-discipline is a principle element that can help.

- **Intermittent fasting is never ending**: Here's another myth; some people have themselves and others believe that once you begin an intermittent fast, you have to keep it going for life. Now to these sets of people, I would love to ask the straightforward question; "What was the purpose of the fast in the first place?" To burn up a lot of calories and mostly achieve weight loss, not so? Now this eating plan being effective is seeing that the desired result has been achieved. Once the desired results have been seen, there is no need to continue with the exercise. All you need to do from then is watch what you eat, so you won't get excessive calories stored up again. Intermittent fasting helps you train your taste buds to loathe foods with a high percentage of calories; you don't have to struggle to abstain from them anymore after staying through to the intermittent fasting plan for you.

These myths do not clamp down the efficacy of the intermittent fasting method. Logically and ideally, intermittent fasting has more health and metabolic benefits than can be seen. Maybe they just choose to ignore the positives and center on the negatives. The benefits of Intermittent fasting even over very short terms cannot be over-emphasized. Fasting exposes the body to a lot of beneficial processes that bulky calories would not let it access. Gene expressions, metabolic waste removal processes, the formation of new neurons and Cellular repair are some of these beneficial processes that go on in the body during fasting to mention, but a few.

Chapter 4 Pros and Cons of Intermittent Fasting

The Different dietary examples have gotten consideration as an approach to reach and keep up a solid weight and pick up well-being benefits even in effectively sound people.

Research is progressing to comprehend the upsides and downsides of intermittent fasting completely. Long haul contemplates are missing to know without a doubt if this eating style gives enduring advantages

Pros

Simple to Follow

Numerous dietary examples center around eating specific nourishments and restricting or keeping away from different food sources. Learning the particular standards of an eating style can require a significant time duty. For instance, there are whole books committed to understanding the DASH diet or figuring out how to follow a Mediterranean-style feast plan. On an eating plan that joins Intermittent fasting, you just eat as indicated by the hour of day or day of the week. When you've figured out which intermittent fasting convention is best for you, all you need is a watch or a schedule to realize when to eat.

No Calorie Counting

As anyone might expect, individuals attempting to reach or keep up a good weight for the most part like to maintain a strategic distance from calorie tallying. While nutrition names are virtually found on numerous nourishments, the way toward estimating segment measures and organizing day by day tallies either physically or on a cell phone application can be dull.

An investigation distributed in 2011 found that individuals are bound to follow plans when all pre-estimated calorie-controlled nourishments are provided.3 Commercial eating diets, WW, Jenny Craig, and others offer these assistance types for a charge. Nonetheless, numerous individuals don't have the assets to pay for these projects, incredibly long haul. Intermittent fasting gives a basic elective where practically no calorie-checking is required. Much of the time, calorie limitation (and along these lines weight loss) happens because nourishment is either wiped out or essentially confined on specific days or during particular hours of the day.

No Macronutrient Limitations

There are well known eating plans that practically confine explicit macronutrients. For instance, numerous individuals follow low-carb eating intend to support wellbeing or get in shape. Others follow a low-fat eating diet for therapeutic or weight loss purposes. Every one of these projects requires the shopper to embrace another eating method—regularly supplanting most loved nourishments with new and perhaps new food sources. This may require new cooking abilities and figuring out how to shop and unexpectedly stock the kitchen.

None of these abilities are required when intermittent fasting. There is no objective macronutrient extend and no macronutrient is limited or taboo.

Unrestricted Eating

Any individual who has ever changed their eating routine to accomplish a health advantage or arrive at a stable weight realizes that you begin to desire nourishments that you are advised not to eat. Indeed, an investigation distributed in 2017 affirmed that an expanded drive to eat is critical during a weight loss venture.

In any case, this test is explicitly constrained on an Intermittent Fasting plan. Nourishment limitation just happens during certain restricted hours. On the non-fasting hours or days of the arrangement, you can by and large eat anything you desire. Specialists here and there call nowadays "devouring" days.

Proceeding to eat undesirable nourishments may not be the most promising approach to pick up profits by Intermittent fasting, however, removing them during specific days constrains your general intake and may at last give benefits.

Might Boost Longevity

One of the most broadly referred advantages of intermittent fasting includes life span. As indicated by the National Institute on Aging, rat examines have demonstrated that when mice are put on projects that seriously confine calories (regularly during fasting periods) many showed an augmentation of life expectancy and diminished paces of a few ailments, particularly malignant growths.

So does this advantage reach out to people? As per the individuals who advance the eating diets, it does. Nonetheless, long haul contemplates are expected to affirm the advantage. As indicated by a survey distributed in 2010, there have been observational research connecting strict fasting too long haul life span benefits. Yet, it was difficult to decide whether fasting gave the advantage or whenever related variables had an impact.

Advances Weight Loss

In a survey of intermittent fasting research distributed in 2018, creators report that the examinations they inspected indicated a massive diminishing in fat mass among subjects who took an interest in clinical preliminaries. They also saw that intermittent fasting was productive in decreasing weight, regardless of the weight list. In any case, it is conceivable that IF is not any more potent than conventional calorie limitation. Intermittent fasting might be not any more compelling than different weight control plans that confine calories all the time. A recent report contrasted intermittent fasting and customary eating diets (characterized as constant energy limitation) and found that weight loss benefits are comparable. It is likewise conceivable that weight loss results may rely upon age. An examination distributed in the diary Nutrition in 2018 inspected the impacts of intermittent fasting (time-limited benefiting from) youthful (20-year-old) versus more established (50-year-elderly people) men. Intermittent fasting somewhat diminished weight in the young, however not in the more established men. Nonetheless, muscle power remained the equivalent in the two gatherings.

Glucose Control

In 2018, some intermittent fasting specialists recommend that this eating style may help those with type 2 diabetes oversee glucose. In any case, the discoveries have been conflicting.

Nonetheless, another investigation distributed in 2019 indicated a less fantastic effect on blood glucose control. Scientists led a two-year follow-up of a year mediation contrasting intermittent fasting and persistent calorie limitation in individuals with type two diabetes. They found that HbA1c levels expanded in both the constant calorie limitation and intermittent gatherings at two years. These discoveries were reliable with results from different investigations demonstrating that notwithstanding a scope of dietary mediations it isn't unprecedented for blood glucose levels to increment after some time in those with type 2 diabetes. The examination creators do note, notwithstanding, that Intermittent energy limitation might be better than ceaseless energy limitation for keeping up lower HbA1c levels, yet noticed that more investigations are expected to affirm the advantage.

Cons

Side Effects

Studies exploring the advantages of Intermittent fasting also point to specific symptoms during the eating program's fasting phase.

For instance, it isn't remarkable to feel irritable, tired, and experience cerebral pains when your calories are minimal. Almost certainly, these reactions will happen when nourishment is altogether dispensed with (for instance, during programs like substitute day fasting) and more averse to happen when nourishment intake is diminished, (for example, on the 5:2 eating diet when 500–600 calories are devoured during fasting days).

Decreased Physical Activity

One eminent reaction of intermittent fasting might be the decrease in physical activity. Most Intermittent fasting programs do exclude a suggestion for physical movement. Of course, the individuals who follow the projects may encounter enough exhaustion that they neglect to meet everyday step objectives and may even change their ordinary exercise schedules.

Proceeding with inquiring about has been proposed to perceive how intermittent fasting may influence physical action designs.

Extreme Hunger

As anyone might expect, it is regular for those in the fasting phase of an IF eating intends to encounter serious appetite. This craving may turn out to be increasingly outrageous when they are around other people who are devouring common dinners and bites.

Medications

Numerous individuals who take meds locate that taking their solution with nourishment assists with mild specific symptoms. A few meds explicitly convey the proposal that they ought to be taken with nourishment. Hence, taking meds during fasting might be a test.

Any individual who takes drugs ought to address their medicinal services supplier before beginning an IF convention to ensure that the fasting stage won't meddle with the prescription's viability or symptoms.

No Focus on Nutritious Eating

The foundation of most intermittent fasting programs is timing, instead of nourishment decision. Along these lines no nourishments (counting those that need great nutrition) are stayed away from and nourishments that give great nutrition are not advanced. Hence, those following the eating diet don't figure out how to eat a solid eating diet.

May Promote Overeating

During the "devouring" phase of numerous intermittent fasting conventions, feast size and supper recurrence are not limited. Rather, shoppers appreciate a not indispensable eating diet. Sadly, this may advance indulging in certain individuals. For instance, if you feel denied following a day of complete fasting, you may feel slanted to indulge (or eat an inappropriate nourishments) on days when "devouring" is permitted

Long-term Limitations

While intermittent fasting isn't new, a significant part of the examination exploring this eating style's advantages is moderately later. Consequently, it is difficult to discern whether the benefits are durable. Furthermore, specialists regularly remark that long haul considers are expected to decide whether the eating plan is even safe for over a while.

Until further notice, the most secure strategy is to work with your human services supplier when picking and beginning an IF program. Your social insurance group can screen your advancement, including medical advantages and worries to ensure that the eating style is reliable for you.

Chapter 5 Preparation, Reason, Tips and Tricks

While Intermittent Fasting isn't difficult, starting a new diet is always a big change. When to start? What to eat? How to eat?

Track Eating Behaviors

The reason that most diets fail is that most of them calculate a desired daily calorie deficit that is based on your initial weight. As you get slimmer, you require a smaller calorie deficit to lose weight. If you stick to the initial number, you are putting more strain on your body than it needs, so your metabolism slows down. Traditional diets are usually hard to maintain because you have to think about mealtimes and meal planning to make the diet unsustainable. Also, most diets don't address eating habits and particularly habitual and emotional eating.

Your weight gain could have a lot to do with your eating behaviors. Eating beside any other reason than being physically hungry is wrong. You could be eating out of boredom, stress, or to compensate for unfulfilled emotional needs. The best way for you to determine why you are overeating is to track your meals, the reasons you thought you were hungry, and what you ate at that time. This approach will help you identify when, how much, and which foods you eat for the wrong reasons. It will make it easier for you to determine the foods you need when truly physically hungry.

Set Goals

A healthy weight loss goal is to lose between one and two pounds every week. If you start losing more, there's a chance that you are losing muscle mass. There's credible research to confirm that it's possible to lose lean muscle mass with Intermittent Fasting if you don't eat enough protein. You can be healthy when it comes to weight but still have high amounts of abdominal fat, which can cause many health risks. The goals with Intermittent Fasting depend on your health and weight goals. You can determine your diet goals by answering a couple of simple questions:

Which improvements are you seeking? Do you want to:

- *Reduce the symptoms of illness,*
- *Feel better,*
- *Become more energized,*
- *Lose weight, or*
- *All of the above?*

• Are you interested in practicing the diet long-term, or only until you meet your goals?

• How will you track the intake of macronutrients?

- What are your diet preferences?

Calculate Body Mass Index

Body Mass Index or BMI is an indicator of whether your current weight is healthy compared to your height. You can calculate your BMI by dividing your weight in kilograms by your squared height (m). If your results are between 18.5 and 24.9, you are healthy. Anything below 18.5 isn't beneficial. The ideal measure is 21 for women and 23 for men. However, this calculation doesn't account for body fat, waist circumference, eating habits, and lifestyle. All of this goes into how healthy you are.

Your BMI can be higher if you are masculine, which doesn't mean that you should lose weight if you are healthy. You can think of yourself as obese if your BMI is over 30. However, this isn't exclusive to the number because it's possible to have a healthy weight with an unhealthy body fat. These are rough calculations that can cause you to think of Athletic and someone who is thinner but has more body fat as obese. However, calculating your BMI can help you determine your weight loss goals in collaboration with your doctor and a dietitian.

Calculate the Body Fat Percentage

Looking into your body-fat percentage will help you to understand what you should do to lose weight, for example:

- Which method of Intermittent Fasting is the most appropriate?

- Whether or not you want to incorporate the Keto diet in the Intermittent Fasting?

- How much do you need to exercise, and what kind of exercises are necessary?

If you like exercising, Intermittent Fasting will help you lose body fat, but preserve or gain muscle mass. As a result, you may not notice scaling down. However, even if you don't lose weight, but gain muscle mass, you will still look slimmer.

To track how your body fat changes, you can use the body composition scales. These scales help you track how your muscle mass, your hydration, and your body fat change throughout your diet.

Calculate Waist-To-Hip Ratio

The waist-hip ratio or WHR is a more credible measurement because it accounts for your natural body shape. For women, an ideal measure is 0.8, while 0.9 is perfect for men. If your measurements are higher, you should work on your profile.

For calculating the WHR, you can use a tape measure and measure the circumference of the widest part of your hips and your natural waist, which is slightly above your belly button. After that, divide your waist measurement by your hip measurement.

Plan Your Portions

Calculate Basal Metabolic Rate

While measuring meals isn't required with Intermittent Fasting, it is desirable to maintain optimal health levels. To start, you should calculate your basal metabolic rate to find out how many calories you need to keep your weight, and how many you need to lose it.

Calculate the Right Portion Sizes

When calculating portion sizes, keep in mind that 1 gram of nutrients translates to a different amount of calories:

- Fat-9 calories,

- Protein- 4 calories, and

- Carbohydrate-4 calories.

Calculate the Daily Calorie Intake

In general, Intermittent Fasting doesn't require calorie restriction for weight loss. Still, weight loss and other health benefits of fasting will be more significant if you have a controlled daily calorie intake.

What to Expect

For most people starting with Intermittent Fasting, skipping breakfast is one of the most drastic changes. No matter how strange it might feel not to have breakfast, resist the temptation if the meal doesn't fit into your feeding window. Your appetite will be suppressed in the morning, and there's no use of eating if you're not hungry.

While most people don't experience severe hunger while fasting, it is possible to get occasional cravings. This happens because the majority of our eating is habitual. As a result of habitual eating, the balance of the hormones in charge of hunger and satiety is disturbed. The longer you fast, the better will these hormones balance out. As you regain a healthy sense of your body's natural appetite, habitual cravings will decrease.

It's also not recommended to eat late in the evening, despite intense cravings you might feel. Doing so will produce more significant amounts of insulin because insulin is maximally stimulated with eating at this time. If you make dinner your largest meal, you will slow down the weight loss. Your largest meal should be around 3 p.m., while the evening meal should be lighter.

What to Look For

You can choose between numerous Intermittent Fasting variations. Some of the ways to determine the right fasting plan are to consider the following:

- Do you need to eat in the morning, or you can delay your first meal?

- Do you get hungry in the evening?

- Do you feel like you want to fast on certain days, but not the others?

Answering these questions will help you determine whether you want to fast daily or fast a certain number of days during a week and eat as usual during the remainder of the week.

Intermittent Fasting Tricks to make it Work

Here are some tips and tricks for ensuring that you have a successful fast:

- Drink plenty of water– as a woman you should drink 1.5-2 liters per day. Make sure you drink water first thing in the morning.

- To keep your hunger at bay, drink coffee and tea as caffeine is a normal suppressant.

- Stay busy and do meaningful work. The busier you are, the lesser time you will time you will think about food. Get out of your house wherever you can!

- Get your best work finished in the morning because you're going to be the most inspired and have a lot of energy.

- Keep it adjustable for you–the best way to do this is to fast at your speed, as the fast suits with your lifestyle, you're more likely to stick to it. Switch the diets around until you find the right one.

- For at least 3 weeks, give it a good try-don't give up too quickly. This takes your body to adapt that amount of time.

- Use vitamins for your benefit.

- Try to delay the breakfast to see how long it can last. It can provide you with a clear example for the best times to fast and eat.

- Don't mention you're fasting to strangers–the less people you meet, the less' helpful thoughts' you're forced to hear. With you, you're doing this. Don't think about that.

- Don't forget to take advantage of training. Weight training to help build up your body, which in turn increases your metabolism.

- Protein is a friend of yours. When necessary, include it in each meal and also use vitamins to help you out.

- Eat well. Don't eat garbage on your non-fasting days. In the long run, this will discourage you. It is important to remember that the day's first meal will set the tone for the remainder of the day. Make it a good one!

Insider Tips for Breaking a Fast

It's important to know when to stop fasting as it is the key to safety. If you feel 'real hunger', this means you need to listen to body and reading the signals when you're done.

The dictionary describes hunger as "the unpleasant feeling of exhaustion induced by the need for food." If they are not eaten at their regular mealtime, certain people are irritable, nervous, or disoriented. Others have the feeling of hunger as lightheaded, flat, weak, headachy, or hollow. Sometimes a feeding episode is caused by a growling stomach. Many people eat when they become sad. Some, when tired, lose their appetite. External stimuli, as well as emotional and physical stimuli, are plentiful, but few of them are hungry, just another burden on your nervous system.

Other signs it's time to end the fast include:

- Sudden sickness or nausea.

- Diarrhea.

- Rapid increase or decrease in your heart rate.

- Excessive dehydration.

- Sudden excessive weakness.

- Usually, your experience is a great indicator. Often when the time is up, you'll know.

The recovery time for breaking a fast is estimated to be around 4 days. During this time, easy-to-digest food consumption is essential to your whole system in order to get used to the new routine.

Include suggestions for stuff you should consume (start adding new items from the top of the list):

- Fruit and vegetable juices

- Raw fruits

- Vegetable or bone broths

- Yogurt (or other living, cultured milk products), unsweetened

- Lettuces and spinach

- Cooked vegetables and vegetable soups

- Raw vegetables

- Well-cooked grains and beans

- Nuts and eggs

- Milk products (non-cultured)

- Meats and anything else

More tips for breaking a fast successfully:

- Pay attention to the way that your body reacts to these new foods (above). Any adverse reactions are there for a reason.

- Look out for feeling full. Once you reach this, stop eating.

- Start with small, frequent meals. Eat every 2 hours or so, while slowly progressing towards more extensive, more normal sized meals.

- Always chew your food well as this aids digestion.

- Eat carefully to add live enzymes and good bacteria into your body. Fresh, raw foods are a great way to achieve this.

10 Proven Tips for Managing Your Fast

Each segment will cover the practical tips that are needed to manage your days of fasting. If you continue with your intermittent fasting regime, these will benefit you.

1. *When you get hungry, hunger suppressants* help you get through the fasting window when you get thirsty. These include coffee, sugar, green tea, cinnamon and chia seeds. Use these in order to help you get through!

2. *The mixture of diet and exercise:* This is possible; several tests have shown that it's okay! You're going

to work out what time of day is better for your training after a while.

3. *Getting tired or dizzy:* This is usually due to dehydration, so make sure you're drinking plenty. Increasing your salt intake is also advisable– particularly if headaches become a concern.

4. *I'm struggling here:* The best way to avoid giving up is to stay busy. By getting out and doing something constructive, take your mind off food.

5. *I'm too busy:* This can be for your benefit because your focus is not always going to be on food. Prepare a quick that matches the current hours of work / commitments before this becomes troublesome. There's no reason for not doing that–particularly not that.

6. *I'm going to gorge:* Once you've accomplished your fast, assume that it never happened and continue as normal. When time goes by, this will make it easier and the body will be adapted.

7. *Things continue to crop up:* That's why it's essential to prepare. Clearing your calendar with crucial things and adapting will be the same as how effective you are.

8. *Meeting with the negativity:* Not everyone knows the effects of fasting, so it's best to educate those who need to hear about it–relatives, close friends, etc.

Others are going to try to put you off or freak you out, stopping you from setting off.

9. *Maintaining the loss of weight:* The fast is not a quick fix. It's a long-term change in lifestyle that will help you keep the slimmer/healthier image you love. It's also best to eat much better and keep this up all the way.

10. *How* to *keep going:* You need to relax if you feel tired. There's something the body is trying to tell you and you need to listen. That's why it's recommended that you clear your schedule at the outset.

Chapter 6 The Intermittent Fasting Types

There are various ways you could engage in intermittent fasting. These types have been proven to give the same effects that have made people start fasting, and some of these potentials benefits include the loss of weight and fat. Some have also discovered that it helps in reducing the risk of getting some diseases.

These are some of the types that are popular and have been proven to show effectiveness:

1. The 16/8 Method

This involves fasting for a total period of 16 hours in the 24 hours that makes a day.

This method requires a daily fast of 14 hours for women and 16 hours for men. You'll have to limit the times you eat to a total of 8- to 10-hour eating window. With this method, you can incorporate 2 to 3 or more meals in a day.

Martin Berkhan, the famous fitness expert, made this method popular. Some refer to it as the Leangains protocol. It is the most popular because it is almost natural. The hours you skip meals fall under the time you are either sleeping or working. Most people who ignore their breakfast and finish dinner before eight are actually doing the 16-hour protocol, but they don't know that.

Women are advised to fast for 14 to 15 hours because most do better with this short range, and during the fast you have to eat healthy foods during the eating window. The results you want to achieve won't be forthcoming if there's a lot of junk in your food.

You can take water and coffee during the fasting hours as well as other drinks that are noncaloric.

To fast with this method, your last meal should be by 8 p.m. while your first meal should be by 12 p.m.

2. The 5:2 Diet

British journalist Michael Mosley popularized this method. It has also been called the fast diet.

This method requires that you limit the number of calories you consume to only 500 for females and 600 for males two days a week. That means you usually eat for five days and reduce the calories in your diet for two days.

For example, you might eat every day of the week except Tuesday and Thursday to reduce the food you consume. You limit the calories for breakfast to 250 for women and 300 for men while dinner takes the same number of calories as well.

3. Eat-Stop-Eat

This method requires you to do a 24-hour fast either once or twice in a week, whichever one is comfortable for you.

An example is not eating from 7 p.m. to 7 p.m. the next day. That is if you start with dinner on Monday, you don't eat from 7 p.m. Monday to 7 p.m. Tuesday. You can do this once or twice in a week. If it is once, it should be done mid-week, like Wednesday, and if it is twice, it is good if the days are spread apart, e.g., Monday and Thursday.

You can drink water, coffee, and other noncaloric drinks between fasting periods, but solid foods are not allowed. However, it is not advisable to start with this method as it requires a lot of energy for the long hours without food. Start with 16 hours fasting before plunging into the 24 hours fast.

4. Alternate-day Fasting

Most of the health benefits that were revealed are as a result of this method. That is fasting on alternate days.

There are two variations to this method;

a) 24-hour full day fasting every other day. This requires you to eat normally for a day and then fast for the next 24 hours.

b) Eating only a few hundred calories. The alternate-day fasting can be very challenging, and this made the experts devise another plan where you only eat a reduced number of calories every other day.

An example is that when you fast on Monday, you usually eat on Tuesday, fast on Wednesday, and the continue for the rest of the week.

5. The Warrior Diet

This method of fasting was made famous by Ori Hofmekler, another fitness expert.

This diet requires you to fast or eat a small or little chunk of food during the day while consuming a massive meal at night, a typical case of fast and feast later. You eat small amounts of fruits and vegetables during the day and fall back to a huge meal.

The meal is best eaten by 4 p.m. No food must be eaten until the next morning when you continue with fruits and vegetables.

Feast for dinner and fast for the day.

6. Spontaneous Meal Skipping

This is a more natural method than the 16/8 because there's no routine. You just skip meals when convenient.

This can be done on some instances, such as when you are not really hungry or on a journey and can't find suitable food. You can skip these meals.

There's no routine to this method. You can decide to skip your meal anytime, from lunch to dinner to breakfast. Once you don't follow a routine, you are using this method.

These methods, however, are not suitable for every individual, and you don't need to try everything before you know which is ideal for you.

This guide is for women over 50 years old, and these kind of people often lose energy more rapidly than typical younger youths so methods, such as the alternate-day fasting and the eat-stop-eat method, are not suitable for women over fifty because these types and processes require a lot of energy, which these women lack.

The 16/8 is not suitable for every one woman over fifty, but it's a good start if you want to take the fast to another level. There's no magic to it, and no one can tell you what's best for you. You have to discover that yourself.

The spontaneous meal skipping is a great place to start, but the results won't be as fast as the other methods because of the lack of routine.

The best methods, however, are the eat-stop-eat and the 5:2. These two have routines you can follow, but you don't need to stay away from food, only consume small calories. This way, you fast with a routine, and the results will be achieved.

Whichever you decide to use, make sure you consult your doctor to see if intermittent fasting is suitable for you.

Chapter 7 Intermittent Fasting For Weight Loss

Diets and exercise can be important components of women's weight loss, but there are many other factors.

Studies show that everything from sleep quality to stress can significantly impact malnutrition, metabolism, corporal weight, and bowel fat.

1. Refined carbohydrates

Cut down on the refined carbohydrates are thoroughly processed, reducing the amount of fiber and micronutrients in the end product.

These foods spike blood sugar levels, increase starvation and are linked to increased body weight and fat.

Therefore, refined carbs such as white bread, pasta and pre-packaged foods can best be limited. Select bulk goods such as spinach, brown rice, quinoa, buckwheat, and barley.

2. Add resistance training to your routine resistance workout builds muscle and improves stamina.

It is perfect for women over 50, since it increases the amount of calories the body burns. It also helps to protect bone mineral density from osteoporosis.

Lifting weights, using gymnastics or carrying out body-weight exercises are just a few simple ways to start.

3. Drink More Water Drinking more water is an easy and efficient way to minimize weight loss.

According to a small study, the number of calories burned in 30-40 minutes was increased temporarily by 16.9 oz (500 ml) of water.

Studies also show that before a meal drinking water can increase weight loss and reduce the number of calories consumed by about 13 percent.

4. Eat more proteins

Protein Foods such as meat, poultry, meat, eggs, milk and legumes, in particular when they concern weight loss, are an essential part of a healthy diet.

In a small 12-week study, an increase in protein intakes by just 15 percent decreased average daily calory intake by 441 calories, resulting in weight loss of 11 pounds (5 kg).

5. Regular sleep preparation studies suggest that sleep can be as critical as diet and exercise to lose weight.

Many studies relate sleep deprivation with increased body weight and higher ghrelin, the stimulating hormone of hunger.

In fact, one study by women found that sleeping for at least 7 hours per night and improving overall sleep quality increases the likelihood of weight loss by 33%.

6. If you do more aerobic cardio exercise, also known as cardio, increase your heart rate to burn additional calories.

Studies show that adding more cardio to your routine can lead to a significant weight loss, especially when combined with a healthy diet.

At least 20–40 minutes of cardio a day or 150–300 minutes a week for the best results.

7. Using a food journal to track what you are eating is an easy way to take responsibility and make healthier choices.

It also facilitates the counting of calories, which can be an effective weight management strategy.

In addition, a food journal can help you to achieve your goals and could lead to a longer-term loss of weight.

8. Add more fiber to your diet is a popular weight loss technique that can help slow your stomach's emptying and make you feel longer.

Without changing diet or lifestyle, an increase of 14 grams per day in dietary fiber intake was associated with a decrease of 10%

in calorie intake and of 4.2 pounds (1.9 kg) of weights over 3.8 months.

Fruits, vegetables, legumes, nuts, seeds and whole grains can all be enjoyed as part of a balanced diet.

9. **Mindful eating Practice**

A meal that minimizes external distractions during your meal. Try to eat slowly and concentrate on how your meals taste, look, smell and feel.

This method encourages healthier eating habits and is a vital tool to improve weight loss.

Studies show that eating slowly improves feelings of fullness and can reduce daily calories significantly.

10. **The range of balanced, low-calorie snacks is an ideal way to lose weight and keep track of hunger levels between meals.**

Snack Smarter

Use high-protein and fiber snacks to encourage fullness and reduce cravings.

Whole fruit, together with nut butter, hummus vegetables, and Greek yoghurt with nuts, are examples of healthier snacks that can support long-lasting weight loss.

11. Ditch the diet

Although fad diets often promise rapid weight loss, when it comes to your skin and health, they can do more harm than good.

For example, one study in women at school has shown that removing particular foods has increased cravings and excessive consumption of food.

Fad diets can also encourage unhealthy eating habits and lead to yo-yo diets, damaging long-term loss of weight.

12. Squeeze in More Steps

If you're time pressed and cannot complete your workout, it's an easy way to burn extra calories and increase weight loss.

In fact, non-exercise activity is estimated to account for 50% of your body's calories during the whole day.

Taking the stairs instead of the lift, parking outside the entrance, or walking during a lunch break, are some basic techniques for bumping the total number of steps and burning more calories.

13. Setting SMART targets will make it easier to meet your weight loss goals while you are improving.

SMART objectives should be specific, measurable, achievable, relevant and timely. We will hold you accountable and prepare how you can accomplish your goals.

Instead of merely setting a goal to waste 10 pounds, for instance, set a goal of losing 10 pounds in 3 months by keeping a food journal, going to the gym three times a week and adding some vegetables for each meal.

14. Some studies suggest that higher stress levels can contribute to a higher risk of weight gain over time.

Stress may also change eating patterns and lead to problems such as excessive eating and binging.

Training, listening to music, practicing yoga, journaling and communicating with family and friends are several easy and effective ways to reduce stress.

15. Try HIIT High-intensity, also called HIIT, interval training, with intense movement explosions with short recovery times to keep your heart rate high.

Cardio switching for HIIT can increase weight loss several times a week.

HIIT may lower bowel fat, improve weight loss and burn more calories than other activities, such as biking, running and resistance training.

16. Using smaller plates

Switching to a smaller plate size will help to reduce the part, helping to lose weight.

Although research is minimal and inconsistent, one study showed that participants eating less and more satisfied than those using a plate in the standard size ate less and felt more satisfied.

You can also limit your size with a smaller plate, which reduces your risk of overeating and controls your calorie consumption.

17. Take a probiotic supplement

Probiotics are some kind of beneficial bacteria that can be ingested through food or supplements to promote intestinal health.

Studies show that probiotics can facilitate weight loss by rising fat excretion and adjusting hormone levels to lower appetite.

Lactobacillus gasseri is in particular a probiotic strain that is particularly effective. Studies show that belly fat and excess body weight can be decreased.

18. Yoga practice

Yoga practices demonstrate that yoga can help prevent weight gain and improve fat burning.

Yoga can also reduce stress levels and anxiety— both related to emotional eating.

Furthermore, yoga has been shown to reduce binge eating and prevent food concerns to support healthy eating behaviour.

19. Chew Slower

Chewing slowly and fully can help increase weight loss by reducing the amount of food you eat.

According to a study, the intake of chewing 50 times per morsel decreased significantly compared with chewing 15 times per morsel.

Another study showed that chewing food reduces the intake by 9.5% and 14.8% respectively, by either 150 or 200 percent higher than normal.

20. **Enjoy a nutritious breakfast in the morning can help you start your day on the right foot and keep you feeling full up until your next meal.**

Studies show that adherence to a regular food pattern could be associated with a reduced risk of binge eating.

It has been shown that eating a high-protein breakfast decreases the levels of the starving hormone Ghrelin. This can help to control appetite and hunger.

21. **Intermittent fasting requires switching between food and fasting for a specific time period every day.**

Fasting cycles usually last 14–24 hours.

Intermittent fasting is considered as effective as calorie-cutting in weight loss.

It can also contribute to improving metabolism by increasing the calories consumed at rest.

22. The foods processed are usually high in calories, sucrance and sodium— but low in important nutrients such as protein, fiber and micronutrients.

Limit Processed Foods

Studies show that consumption of more processed foods is linked to excess body weight— particularly among women.

Therefore, it is best to limit your intake of processed foods and choose whole foods, including fruit, vegetables, healthy fats, magnetic proteins, whole grains, and legumes.

23. Sugar is a major contributor to weight gain and serious health problems such as diabetes and heart disease.

Foods high in additional sugar are full of extra calories. They lack the vitamins, minerals, fiber and protein your body needs to thrive.

Therefore, it is best to limit the intake of sucrant food such as soda, candy, fruit juice, sport drinks, and desserts so that weight loss is encouraged and overall health is optimised.

Chapter 8 The Science of
Intermittent Fasting

Understanding the science behind why Intermittent Fasting works will help you to feel confident and comfortable as you change your diet and lifestyle to accommodate this new regime. We will begin by answering the question, *what is autophagy,* before moving on to more specific aspects of this interesting cellular process in the body.

What Is Autophagy?

Autophagy is a process that happens within the human body that has been going on without our knowledge since the beginning of humans. It is only recently that people have begun to harness this process to achieve desired positive results through changes in their diet, such as Intermittent Fasting. We will look at this topic in-depth throughout this book, but here we will begin by looking at what exactly Autophagy is.

Autophagy, as a word, can be broken up into two individual parts. Each of these parts on its own is a separate Greek word—the word auto, which means *self* and the word phagy, which means *the practice of eating.* Putting these together gives you *the practice of self-eating,* which is essentially what autophagy is. This may sound a little intimidating. Still, it is a very natural process that our cells practice all the time without us being any the wiser. Autophagy is the body's way of cleaning itself out.

Essentially, the body has housekeepers that keep everything neat and tidy. Scientists who have been studying this for some time are not beginning to understand that there are ways to manipulate this process within your body in order to achieve things such as weight loss, improved health, reduction of disease symptoms, and so on. This is what we will spend the rest of the book looking at, but first, we will dive into the science of Autophagy a little more.

How Does Autophagy Work?

The process of autophagy involves small "hunter" particles that go around your body, looking for cells or cell components that are old and damaged. The hunter particles then take these cell components apart, getting rid of the damaged parts and saving the useful parts to make new cells later. These hunter cells can also use useful leftover parts to create energy for the body.

Autophagy has been found to happen in all organisms that are multi-cellular, like animals and plants, in addition to humans. While the study of these larger organisms and how autophagy works in their cells is lesser-known, more studies are being done on humans and how diet changes can affect their body's autophagy.

The other function that autophagy serves is that it helps cells to carry out their death when it is time for them to die. There are times when cells are programmed to die because of several different factors. Sometimes these cells need assistance in their death, and autophagy can help them with this or can help to clean up after their death. The human body is all about life and death. These processes are continually going on without our knowledge to keep us healthy and in good form.

As I mentioned, the autophagy process has been going on inside of us for many, many years, since the beginning of humans. This process has been kept around inside our bodies because of the many benefits it can provide us with. It is also essential for our bodies' health, as being able to get rid of waste and damaged parts that are no longer useful to us is essential to our health. If we could not get rid of damaged or broken cells, these damaged particles would build up and eventually make us sick. Our bodies are extremely efficient in everything that they do, and waste disposal is no different.

In more recent years, the study of autophagy has been focused more heavily on in terms of diet and disease research. These studies are still in their early stages as it has been only a few years shy of sixty years since autophagy was discovered. This process was discovered in a lab by testing what happened when small organisms went without food for some time. These organisms were observed very closely under a microscope. It was found that their cells had this process of waste disposal and energy creation that was later named autophagy.

More about autophagy and its relation to energy production is being studied in recent years, as this topic is interesting to humans. Autophagy can use old cell parts and recycle them to create new energy that the organism (like the human or animal) can use to do its regular functions like walking and breathing. Now, people are studying what happens when humans rely on this form of energy production instead of the energy they would get from ingesting food throughout the day. This is where autophagy and intermittent fasting come together. We will look at how they work together throughout the rest of this book as we delve deeply into intermittent fasting and autophagy and how they work together to allow for things like weight loss or disease prevention.

What Does Autophagy Do?

Autophagy has many functions in the body. In this section, we will look at some of the other autophagy functions and the body systems involved.

Autophagy is said to be the housekeeping function of the body. If you think of your body as your home, autophagy is the housekeeper that you hire to take care of all of the waste and the recycling functions of your cells.

One of the housekeeping duties includes removing cell parts that were built wrongly or at the wrong time. Sometimes cells make mistakes, and these mistakes can cause proteins or other cell parts to be formed in error. When this happens, we need something within the cell to get rid of these so that they do not take up space or get in the way of other processes within the cell. Further, sometimes useful parts of the cell will become damaged somehow and then will need to be removed in order to make way for a new part to take its place. These cell parts can include those that create DNA or those that create the proteins needed to make the DNA.

Another duty of autophagy is to protect the body from disease and pathogens. Pathogens are bacteria or viruses that can infect our cells and our bodies if they are not properly defended. Autophagy works to kill the cells within our body infected by these pathogens to get rid of them before they can spread. In this way, autophagy plays a part in our immune system. It acts as a supplement to our immune cells whose sole function is to protect us from disease and infection invasions.

Autophagy also functions to help the body's cells regulate themselves when there are stressors placed upon them. These stressors can be things like a lack of food for the cell or physical stresses placed on the cell. This regulation helps to maintain a standard cell environment despite factors that can change, like food availability. Autophagy is able to do things like break down cell parts for food to provide the cell with nutrients.

Similar to its role in regulating the cells, autophagy also helps with the development of a growing fetus inside a woman's uterus. Autophagy occurs here to ensure that the embryo has enough nutrients and energy at all times for healthy development. In addition to this, it helps with growth in adults and there is a balance of building new parts and breaking down old ones involved in the growth of any organism.

Autophagy is more important than we may even realize, as it plays a large role in the survival of the living organisms it acts within. It does this by being especially sensitive to the levels of nutrients and energy within a cell. When the nutrient levels lower, autophagy breaks down cell parts, creating nutrients and energy for the cell. If it weren't for this process, the cells would not be able to maintain their ideal functioning environment. They may begin to make more mistakes and even lower their functioning abilities altogether. So much goes on inside a cell that they need to work effectively at all times. Autophagy makes this possible, which is what makes it such an essential function.

Using Intermittent Fasting to Induce Autophagy

Autophagy functions in the following way. When a decrease in nutrients is noticed within a cell, this decrease in nutrients acts as a signal for the cell to create small pockets within a membrane (a thin barrier layer) called *autophagosomes*. These small pockets (autophagosomes) move through the cell and find debris and damaged particles floating around within the cell. The small pockets then consume this debris by absorbing it into its inner space. The debris is then enclosed in the membrane (the thin barrier layer) and is moved to a place in the cell called the Lysosome. A lysosome is a part of a cell that acts as a center for degradation, breakdown, or disassembly. This part of the cell gets debris and damaged cell parts delivered to it by the autophagosomes. Once these damaged cell parts are delivered, the lysosomes then break them down. By breaking them down, these parts can be recycled and used for energy.

The most common way to induce autophagy in a person is by way of starvation. This is not to say that a person must starve themselves, but they starve their cells of nutrition temporarily. This is why people turn to fasting to induce autophagy. Low nutrition levels within the cells is the most common way that autophagy is triggered, as it is a process that creates energy within the cell. By knowing this, scientists have concluded that by inducing starvation within the cells, one can intentionally upregulate autophagy in their body. Intermittent Fasting involves periods of fasting, which then induces a state of starvation within the cells (simply meaning that there is no energy being consumed to use for energy) and so it induces autophagy in the cells to make energy.

Other Ways to Induce Autophagy

Starvation

The most common way to induce autophagy in a person is by way of starvation. Autophagy is triggered by a decrease in nutrients within a cell. As I mentioned above, this decrease in nutrients acts as a signal within the cell to begin autophagy, which is exactly how Intermittent Fasting works.

Aerobic Exercise

One other way to activate autophagy is through exercise. Aerobic exercise has been shown through studies to increase autophagy in the cells of the muscles, the heart, the brain, lungs, and the liver.

Sleep

Sleep is very important for autophagy. If you have ever gone a few days without a proper, restful sleep, you know that you begin to feel a decline in your mental abilities rather quickly. This could be because of your brain's decreased autophagy functioning. The number of hours that you are in bed does not matter if the sleep is not good quality, though. Quality sleep for the right number of hours is what is needed to maintain good brain function and keep your brain's autophagy going.

Specific Foods

The consumption of specific foods has been shown to induce or promote autophagy. The added benefit is that not only do they trigger autophagy in the cells of your body, these foods are also shown to have numerous other health benefits.

Chapter 9 Reasons You Should Start Intermittent Fasting Today If You're A Woman over 50

Being a woman is one thing. Being a woman over the age of 50 is another. With age slowly creeping in on you, your body begins to experience some changes. If you are self-aware and alert, you will notice these changes early enough. If you aren't, however, it will likely take a while.

At age 50 and over, it naturally becomes more challenging to shed weight. This is because metabolism will decrease, joints might be more prone to ache, muscle mass will decrease, and you might even experience sleep issues. In addition to these, you'll become more at risk of developing certain age-related diseases and health conditions.

Some of the changes your body will experience might be subtle. Still, they are nonetheless veiled threats to a fully functional body system and definitely to the longevity we all seek.

This is why it is imperative to seek out measures, lifestyles, and diets that could help you lose fat, especially dangerous belly fat. Losing fat will reduce drastically the risks of developing health issues, such as diabetes, heart attack, and cancer.

Below are a few reasons you need to consider intermittent fasting seriously:

Weight Loss

A very high percentage of people who are currently into intermittent fasting did so because they either want to guard against piling up excess body fat or because they want to lose weight. That makes weight loss a primary reason women over the age of 50 should consider giving intermittent fasting a try.

Intermittent fasting generally helps boost metabolism in the body by promoting thermogenesis or production of heat. This will lead to excess body fat being burned and used to fuel the body's activities.

Another way intermittent fasting can help solve weight is by reducing hunger. Thus, the stomach will always have the illusion of being filled.

Weight loss becomes even more natural when the keto diet is combined with intermittent fasting. They both complement each other.

Muscle and Joint Health

Research efforts also proved that intermittent fasting could help women over 50 improve their muscle and joint health. Some of the researchers discovered that the fasting period affects the way the body produces hormones. This will help strengthen the bones and forestall against things like arthritic symptoms and lower back pain.

Intermittent Fasting Can Help To Prevent Cancer

Women over 50 are at risks of developing some kinds of cancer. Intermittent fasting, as shown in research, can cut off some of the pathways leading to cancer. Intermittent fasting can also help slow down the rate at which an existing tumor grows in the body.

Intermittent Fasting and Mental Health

Because of the body changes, the hormonal imbalance, and the uncertainty surrounding the state of things, it could be a mentally disturbing period for women over 50.

The results of a 2018 study showed that women who practiced intermittent fasting reported improvement in moods and self-esteem while anxiety and depression levels dropped.

If you are prone to depression and anxiety disorders, intermittent fasting might just be the easiest way out. But you have to speak with your medical professional first.

Intermittent Fasting Helps with Sleep and Clarity

Hormonal changes in the body can cause one's sleeping pattern to be destabilized, especially around the post-menstrual age.

It is soothing to discover that many older women have testified how the intermittent fasting lifestyle has improved their sleeping patterns.

If you're currently experiencing sleep issues, intermittent fasting is definitely an option for you.

Intermittent Fasting and Longevity

Perhaps the greatest bane of growing older is that old age opens up the body to more risk of developing diseases.

Ultimately, intermittent fasting became so popular among women aged 50 and older because it evidently helps them live longer and in good health.

Some even say it was tailor-made for older women.

Intermittent Fasting Boosts Productivity

Growing old can be quite a boring stage of life for people struggling with their health each day. It could rob them of the joy of living, experiencing life, and getting things done.

Older people are happier when they can stay fit and healthy. While it might be retirement age, there are a lot of things you might want to do with your life at that point, activities that could bring you fulfilment if you're healthy enough to partake in them.

Intermittent fasting helps you experience a boost in productivity by helping to keep you fit and in good health.

In summary, intermittent fasting is the answer to many of the adverse effects of growing older. It keeps you in charge of your body and teaches you how to get the best out of your body system, effectively maximizing your potential to remain in good health for as long as possible.

All you have to do is to ensure that you pick the right fasting method. You might need to pair it with a diet, keto probably. You would also need to discuss this with your doctor/dietitian/psychologist to ascertain what is truly right for you and what is not. Women over 50 cannot afford to take certain health risks. So you have to be sure you can trust your health and wellness regime.

Chapter 10 Intermittent Fasting and Hormones

For women over 50 several hormones come into play by this age. Some of these hormones are reduced while we age, while others are overly active. Intermittent fasting can help you regulate each of these hormones to their optimum. Let's see how each hormone gets affected or reacts through intermittent fasting techniques.

Food and Appetite Hormones

We have seen the effects of intermittent fasting on insulin and how it helps counter insulin resistance. Let's now see how intermittent fasting can help another resistance phenomenon known as the Leptin Resistance. Leptin as we know is the satiety hormone, it tells us we have had enough food and need to stop. But due to various eating disorders and hormonal changes in our body, our brain stops listening to leptin telling us to stop. Though leptin is secreted at the normal levels and is actively present in the bloodstream, our body fails to recognize that it is full and there is no further need for food.

This disorder leads to more and more consumption of food and naturally leads to abnormal weight gains. Intermittent fasting can help you counter leptin resistance. When you are fasting regularly, you are gaining a sense of self control and denying the twisted signals of the hunger hormone. Through continued intermittent fasting you will be able to pass up a plate of cake or your favorite chocolate ice cream without falling into the urge of taking a bite. Because your brain was refusing to listen to normal levels of leptin, your body was producing it in high amounts which still went ignored. But through intermittent fasting, you will be able to scale down your leptin levels making you highly sensitive to even small levels of this hormone. This is what will make you feel full when you have had a good meal. Eating more fiber-rich foods, and low-carb diets can be crucial in this scenario.

The hunger hormone, ghrelin also undergoes considerable changes during fasts. These changes have been known to have positive effects on dopamine levels which in turn improve concentration and cognitive abilities.

Female Reproductive Hormones

Estrogen and Progesterone are the female hormones responsible for various reproductive functions. For women who are younger and still in childbearing age, or menstruating age, intermittent fasting has varying effects. For some women intermittent fasting has been known to be great and non-inhibitory in terms of their reproductive hormones, while for other women who were too sensitive to intermittent fasting, it can also result in disturbed periods or temporary infertility. But, for women who are over the age of 50 this concern disappears as these women no longer produce much estrogen and are beyond the menstruating age. Therefore, period irregularity or infertility are no longer a concern.

A healthy brain-ovary axis is what determines the health of a woman concerning the female hormones. For women over 50, intermittent fasting helps maintain a healthy brain-ovary axis to ensure good hormone health without the concerns of disturbing these hormones.

Even for those who have not yet crossed menopause, intermittent fasting is not risky at all. It all comes down to how you introduce intermittent fasting to your body. Taking things slowly is essential. As your body gets accustomed to smaller fasting periods you can gradually move to longer fasts. Research shows that all the hormonal irregularity occurs when you send your body into shock through fasting for longer periods suddenly. Give yourself and your body sufficient time to get acclimatized to the concept of fasting and you wouldn't need fear any hormonal imbalance due to your fasts.

Adrenal Hormones

Adrenal hormones are the hormones released by the adrenal glands. The adrenal glands are situated over the kidneys. They are responsible for regulating our moods in times of stress, anxiety, and excitement. Of these hormones the most important is the stress hormone, also known as cortisol. A healthy adrenal-brain axis or the hpa axis is necessary to have regulated levels of adrenal hormones. When this balance is disturbed, cortisol levels spike up irregularly or go too low. This is observed to happen with intermittent fasting for longer durations of time. Cortisol levels may swing dangerously to either extreme, increasing the stress levels in our body. This leads to a condition that is commonly known as adrenal fatigue. Most common symptoms of adrenal fatigue are tiredness, muscle weakness, extreme nervousness, sleep issues, and digestive problems.

The HPA axis disturbance can give rise to several circadian rhythm issues. People who are already suffering from circadian rhythm problems find intermittent fasting for prolonged periods highly stressful. For these people it is highly recommended to follow the crescendo method of fasting. Taking it slowly and increasing your fasting hours gradually can be the key to having well-regulated cortisol levels to keep stress at bay.

Thyroid Hormones

It consists of two lobes on either side of the throat, connected by a small bridge like tissue. When thyroid function is normal, it is nearly impossible to feel your thyroid by physical examination. In conditions such as hypothyroidism and Hashimoto's, which is an autoimmune thyroid issue, very often the thyroid is easily felt.

Research has shown that intermittent fasting that included fasting hours during the night and the eating window during the day, had positive improving effects on hypothyroid problems. The thyroid gland is controlled and regulated by the body's internal biological clock known as the circadian rhythm. Keeping the circadian rhythm functioning normally is essential to having normal thyroid functions. Therefore, if the fast can be so observed so as not to disturb the body's inherent biological clock, then it can work in the favor of those suffering from thyroid issues.

It was observed that when the fast was elongated beyond the 16-hour mark, the circadian rhythms were disturbed, and this affected the proper functioning of the thyroid gland in those suffering from hypothyroidism. Longer fasts of around 24 hours or more are highly inappropriate for patients with dysfunctional thyroid activity. Therefore, for hypothyroid patients it is advisable that they fast only for 14 to 16 hours and make it a point to have their eating window during the day. This will help balance their thyroid functioning and regulate their already irregular thyroid hormone levels.

Chapter 11 Best Exercise to Lose Weight after 50 Years Old

At 50, the topic of losing weight and fitness comes to the fore. As estrogen levels drop, the risk of accumulating pounds increases. By reducing the production of sex hormones during menopause, the body's energy requirements decrease and the basal metabolism decreases.

The growth hormone somatotropin, which helps build muscle, is also released less and less. This factor is associated with problems such as changes in body composition, muscle mass is lost, fat tissue builds up from 40 years of age. The metabolism slows down, which also reduces the calorie requirement.

From the age of 50, an almost daily, but shorter workout is recommended to lose weight. Joint-friendly sports such as aqua fitness, swimming or cycling are suitable for boarding. You can also start with 50 new sports: gentle yoga, tai chi, Nordic walking or even climbing. Since the age of 50 there is a risk of redistribution of body fat (more belly fat, less rounding on the hips and buttocks), targeted training on equipment is recommended to build muscle where fat is to be distributed. It is best to have special exercises shown during an introductory training session in the gym.

To keep your weight down, make it easy for yourself and incorporate more exercise into your everyday life. Think about what habits you can change. The classic: climbing stairs instead of an elevator. If your joints and back allow it, you should do your shopping on foot: carrying half an hour of bags consumes around 140 calories. If you don't want to drag, take the bike. Car and bus should be off limits for shorter distances anyway. Gardening is also a good program against flab. Raking half an hour of leaves burns about 160 calories. Or complete a moderate exercise program with walking or walking every day.

Fitness exercise suitable for women over 50

Depending on your physical condition, all types of jogging, walking, swimming, cycling or hiking are highly recommended as endurance sports. Healthy training for the cardiovascular system can, of course, also be done easily indoors, for example on the cross trainer or rowing machine, in special fitness courses or online at home.

During endurance sports, high stress peaks due to possible cardiovascular diseases are to be avoided urgently. In cases of doubt, it is advisable to exercise with a heart rate monitor in order to remain in the optimal, healthy heart rate range.

Small devices such as Thera bands are very suitable for strength training, they offer optimal safety for the joints and can also be used wonderfully at home or on the go.

In addition to endurance and strength training, it is also important to train the coordination and associated control of the body's proprioceptors. Position, sense of movement, strength and balance can be trained and improved through targeted exercises. Exercises such as the one-legged stand serve, among other things, to prevent falls.

Incidentally, physical training also improves mental fitness through improved oxygen supply and the perceptual and cognitive challenge.

Four exercises to keep fit for women 50 years and above

Strengthen leg muscles

Stand next to a chair and hold on to the backrest. With the upper body upright and without kinking at the waist, raise the knee as far as possible towards the chest (if the hip is artificial, lift the thigh at most to the horizontal), slowly lower the leg again and repeat the exercise with the other leg.

Execution: Two series with ten repetitions per leg, always alternating between the left and right leg (so count to 20). In order to intensify the exercise, weight cuffs can also be put on above the ankles; a kilo is enough to start with.

Strengthen hips

Stand behind a chair and hold on to the backrest. Move one leg straight to the side without bending your waist or knees. The toes point forward during the movement. Slowly move the leg back to the starting position and repeat the exercise with the other leg.

Execution: Two series with ten repetitions per leg, always alternating between the left and right leg (count to 20). To increase the effect, weight cuffs can also be put on above the ankles.

Strong upper arms

Sit upright on the front half of the chair surface. Grip the armrests of the chair so that your hands are right next to your torso. Put your feet forward. If possible, push your body up with your arms only, stretching your elbows as far as possible. Slowly sink back into the chair, trying to slow the movement with your arms. Take a deep breath and repeat the exercise.

Execution: Two series with ten repetitions each (with both arms at the same time).

For feet and calf muscles

Stand upright behind a chair and hold on to the backrest. Push your heels off the floor so that you stand on tiptoe. Slowly return to the starting position until the feet are firmly on the floor. Then lift both toes of your feet so that you stand on your heels.

Execution: two to three series with ten to 20 repetitions on both legs or ten repetitions each with one leg. Tip: Gradually increase up to 20 reps. If you find this too easy, try to lift your body weight only on the right or left leg.

Chapter 12 The Healthy Foods to Eat When On the Intermittent Fasting Lifestyle

The foods eaten by an individual who lives with the intermittent fasting lifestyle is a sufficient and balanced diet that allows the individual to sustain their health and weight loss. Their food intake is specific and healthy foods that support their intermittent fasting to maintain functional health status.

An individual who indulges in intermittent fasting should eat more of high fibre foods, such as nuts, beans, fruits and vegetables, and high content foods with protein, including meat, fish, beans, or nuts during the intermittent fasting. An individual that also chews gum high in fibre also helps in the process of sustaining good health. Drinking lots of water during the periods of intermittent fasting helps a lot. Some individuals tend to think they are always hungry whereas they are just thirsty.

For those individuals who drink black coffee or tea or cinnamon or liquorice herbal tea, these beverages, according to researchers, tend to have appetite-suppressing effects.

A certified dietitian will help you create the best intermittent fasting eating plan, making sure you don't waste your fasting efforts.

Water is an essential element required for the sustainable growth and healthy living of an individual. Coffee is another element an individual who undergoes intermittent fasting can drink for a healthy living. The question among new intermittent fasters is whether coffee works, or can they take coffee when they indulge in the intermittent fasting? Coffee is naturally a calorie-free beverage. It can be consumed even outside your chosen meal window. Yet, coffee intake can be potentially threatening to the intermittent fasting lifestyle. This is because coffee drinkers rarely drink it without any of creamers, syrups, flavorings, and the likes. Habitual coffee drinkers need to be careful if they wish to enjoy the intermittent lifestyle's full benefits.

Minimally processed grains, which are carbohydrates in nature, are also essential. Carbs aren't harmful to your intermittent fasting lifestyle, and they constitute an integral part of our nutrition. During this diet, it is crucial to note the strategic ways of having enough calories.

Lentils are essential foods that are essential for fitness and check of weight. Lentils contain a very high concentration of fibre and provide you with the right amount of grain needed. Lentils also help you accumulate the required amount of iron, an important nutrient for your body, most especially for a woman practicing the intermittent fasting lifestyle. This could represent about 15 percent of your body's daily iron needs.

Potatoes are another kind of food that is truly beneficial to individuals on the intermittent fasting lifestyle. Like bread, they are particularly easy to digest, requiring no major effort on the body's part. When combined with a source of protein, they are easily the best pairing to consume after a workout session. This is because they help to refuel your hungry muscles. One other benefit attached to potatoes is that they can evolve into starch to feed the good bacteria in your body, once cooled.

Salmon is also a very rich protein source. It is amongst the most common foods in many parts of the world. Salmon is a major factor in the production of omega-3, a couple of fatty acids known as DHA and EPA.

Soybeans help to induce cell damage and promote anti-ageing among human development and growth stage.

Multivitamins are also elements that assist in boosting an individual's health who is into intermittent fasting. Although they will never be direct replacements for a balanced diet containing a healthy amount vegetables, supplements can come in handy during the period of intermittent fasting.

Another element that allows for good health in intermittent fasting is vitamin D fortified milk. Adults are required to take 1,000 milligrams of calcium or about 3 cups of milk per day. Since the allocated time for feeding is low, keeping up with this may prove not very easy, so it is essential to get more calcium than ever. Taking milk helps provide the body with enough calcium and keep the bones active. To make sure your calcium level remains high, you can add milk to your smoothies or cereal or drink it with meals. To ensure your calcium composition remains on the high side, you might want to make milk a regular addition to your cereals or smoothies.

Blueberries might be quite tiny in size, but that does not do justice to how beneficial they are on your intermittent fasting journey. Studies have revealed that longevity and youthfulness are by-products of the anti-oxidative process aided by blueberries, especially the wild variety. It has been proven by research that by aiding the body's anti-oxidative process, wild blueberries keep your youthfulness and increase longevity. As antioxidants, they also help your body's cellular damage in mass quantities.

Papaya, a fruit, can be taken in large quantities by women undergoing intermittent fasting to boost their health status.

Papaya is also imperative in boosting the health status of an individual who undergoes intermittent fasting. As your fast winds down to the final few hours, you may likely begin to experience the effects of going through that number of hours without food. Because of this, you might overeat. The resultant effect of which is sluggishness and bloating. A distinct enzyme in papaya called papain can help ease break down protein in the body, making the digestive process easier and any bloat more manageable.

Many more healthy foods improve health status during intermittent fasting apart from the ones listed and explained above. Without excluding any variety, nuts can also help your longevity.

So, making the right choice of food during your fasting period is entirely up to you.

Chapter 13 Tips to Successful Intermittent Fasting

This chapter is all about helping you make your life easier when it comes to implementing intermittent fasting. There are a few pitfalls that a lot of beginners fall into and following these tips will help you avoid them.

Let's first take a look at the IF side of things.

Intermittent Fasting Tips

These tips will help you get adjusted to IF quickly once you begin.

Drink Water

I've mentioned this before but it bears repeating. Dehydration is something that can derail you off your path pretty quickly. Your body will let go of any excess water it holds in the beginning and you will see a drop in weight. Don't mistake this for fat loss however, it's just water weight.

Despite this water being considered unnecessary, such a sudden release of fluid can trigger dehydration in some people. The thing to do is to play it safe and prevent it from the start. Purchase a water bottle that has markings on it so you know how much water you're drinking throughout the day.

Aim to drink slightly more than your required intake level and monitor yourself for the symptoms of dehydration. Keep in mind that exercise will result in water loss and you should replenish this water as much as possible. You might be tempted to think that energy drinks will do the job but remember that they contain a lot of sugar and aren't the best option for you.

Stick to good ol' water and you'll be fine.

Plan Ahead

Take some time the night before to plan your day ahead. When will your fasting window end and will you be able to eat a meal at that time? When will you cook and do you need to prep. Prepping is something that tends to catch people out for the most part. This is mostly due to it being a habit they haven't practiced before.

Either way, adopt a preventive approach to all the things you need to do and plan everything out. During the day, try to stay active and busy with tasks. This will keep your mind away from food and hunger. The first few times you carry out IF, you will feel hungry.

Remember that this isn't your body feeling hungry. It's simply a reaction to it expecting food then thanks to the way it has been conditioned. In other words, it's clock hunger and isn't real. You can try to drink some water at this time or have a cup of coffee to push it back. Over the course of a week, you'll find that your body will adjust to it and you'll be fine.

Use Coffee and Tea

When clock hunger strikes your best friends will be coffee and tea. Tea is an especially good choice, specifically green tea. Green tea is a great source of antioxidants and helps fight free radicals. Over and above this, drinking fluids helps reduce those hunger pangs that will occur during the first week when you're adopting IF.

Combine IF With Other Protocols

One of the best things you can do once you've adjusted to IF is to combine it with a low carb diet such as the ketogenic diet. This will help you lose fat a lot faster. Keep in mind that the keto diet is not an easy one to follow, especially for vegans. The best approach to take is to ease into it.

You can start by following it on your rest days to see if you're able to make it work. If this is the case, you can expand it to your workout days. Your body will take some time to adjust to the keto diet. To be honest, the diet itself is the subject of an entire book and in the interest of space, I'll restrict myself to a few important points.

The first thing to remember with keto is that your body is going to take some time to adjust from burning carbs to fat. Remember that carbs are the primary fuel source and your body isn't going to flip a switch and start burning fat simply. There is a transition period and this often referred to as the keto fog.

During this time, which lasts for a week or so, you will feel less energized and you'll feel as if you're not able to get out of second gear. The fog lasts for a week and once this time passes, your body will be able to burn fat as its primary source of fuel pretty easily. Practicing keto on your non-training days is a good way to get your body used to burning fat as its primary fuel source.

The best way to prepare for keto is to plan ahead of time and make sure your meal prep is on point. Always start with your protein intake and then move to the other macros. It is best to calculate your macros and calories upfront and then keep your meals as uniform as possible to avoid calorie counting becoming overwhelming.

Ease yourself into keto much as you would with IF and you'll find that both protocols combined will make a massive difference to your overall health.

Do Not Binge

A common mistake beginners make is to look at the feeding window's start as being a free for all as far as food is concerned. At first, this can be hard to resist since you'll look at the fasting period as being a wasteland without any food whatsoever. The reason this point of view develops is because people think of IF as being restrictive.

When I say restrictive, I mean that some people think of it as a protocol where you deny yourself food for a period of time and need to use your willpower to stop yourself from eating. Here's the thing: Human beings are well designed to fast. Think of how our ancestors lived before we built cities and farms and gave birth to the Kardashians.

Food was scarce and wasn't guaranteed. After all, there isn't any deer in this world that will willingly offer itself up to be eaten. People had to go through periods where there wasn't any food available and they still managed to survive. We've come to associate the clock with our meal times and more often than not we feel clock hunger and not real hunger.

It's gotten to the point where some people don't even know what hunger feels like. IF is simply bringing you back into your natural eating pattern and is preventing you from going down the rabbit hole of allowing the clock to dictate what your stomach needs.

The other problem is with regards to breakfast. How often has someone wagged their finger at you and said, "Breakfast is the most important meal of the day!" Here's a fun fact for you: That saying was a marketing slogan invented by Kellogg's to sell more cereal. Here's another fun fact: John Harvey Kellogg the founder of the company figured breakfast was the solution to cure the sin of masturbation amongst young people (The Surprising Reason Why Dr. John Harvey Kellogg Invented Corn Flakes, 2020).

No, I'm not making that up! You can see his line of thought. You can't masturbate if you're shoving god awful cereal into your face, can you? Either way, that's the background story of the so called "most important meal of the day". There is no proof of any adverse effects of skipping breakfast or of not eating breakfast during the time designated for it.

All in all, don't worry about skipping breakfast or even a meal. All that matters is your calories in versus out. Recognize what clock hunger is and get back in touch with your body's needs.

Exercise Tips

Here are some tips to make exercising and staying active easier for you. People think of exercise as being a chore and perhaps you're looking at it the same way.

Activity... Not Exercise

If you feel exercise is too darn painful for you to carry out regularly, make it a goal to be as active as possible. Walk as much as you can, climb a flight of stairs instead of taking the elevator and so on. Try lifting your grocery bags instead of using a cart to push them to your car and so on.

One of the best ways to start getting active is to find a community. Don't worry about joining gyms and so on in the beginning. Just start moving and find someone to move with you. A great way to get fit is to join a salsa or a Zumba class where you'll meet other like-minded people and essentially con yourself into getting fit.

These classes only go so far though and once your body adjusts to it, you will need to join a gym to keep building your muscle mass. Again, you're not going to turn into the hulk. There are who knows how many millennia of evolution built into your body and genes and to think that a few weights will turn you into a man is absurd.

Joining a Crossfit Box (gym) is a great way of getting fit. The workout is planned for you and you're guaranteed a community that will support you in your fitness journey. It can be intimidating to join but once you do you'll find that the community aspect is Crossfit's best quality.

The workout will help you build muscle and lose fat and you'll also receive education from the trainers as to the best way to stay fit. In addition to this, one of the problems beginners face at the start is overtraining. Having an instructor around will prevent this from happening.

If you do join a regular gym by yourself, follow the starting strength program. This is a very well structured program that will guide you every step of the way. You'll always know where you stand so don't worry about getting lost.

Progressive Overload

Every exercise you do, remember the principle of progressive overload. This applies to activities that don't involve weights as well. Push yourself a little bit more every single time you perform the activity.

The biggest advantage, aside from better performance, is that you'll discover your boundaries easily. You'll learn how to listen to your body and be able to differentiate between laziness and genuine fatigue. Keep pushing yourself in this manner and your brain will get used to being uncomfortable and expand your limits.

Motivation

Everyone has bad days and there are sometimes when you just need a break from all of it. A break is a great idea but the problem is that most people don't know how to go about doing it at first. The best way to figure out if you need to take a step back is to adopt a 'do something' approach.

Let's say you return from work and don't feel like going to the gym. You feel exhausted and you feel mentally spent. Suit up and go to the gym anyway. Walk on the floor and try to go through your workout. For most beginners, these workouts will be amongst the best they'll ever have. Your brain will try to trick you using laziness. Once you find that you can perform to your usual levels without any issues, you'll be energized and feel refreshed.

Then there are times when you'll find that you genuinely cannot perform the activity in question. In such cases, feel free to pack up and return home. Remember, discipline is great but being kind to yourself is the most important thing. I'm not talking about giving into laziness but to heed genuine concerns. If your body tells you it needs rest and if you confirm this need (via inadequate performance in the gym,) simply go home and call it a day.

Most beginners do the opposite. They give into laziness in the name of listening to their bodies and push through fatigue in the name of being motivated. You already know why you're getting into IF. The very fact that you're reading this book indicates that you have all the motivation you need.

What you think of as a lack of motivation is temporary fatigue or laziness. As you become more experienced and learn to listen to your body, you'll differentiate between the two easily. At the start, do something and you'll understand the differences better.

Change it up!

Your body will get used to the activities you perform when you carry them out over time. Take a week's break from your regularly scheduled activities to perform something else. This will refresh your muscles and give them a different challenge to deal with. For example, if you're on Starting Strength and want to switch things up, suspend the program for a week.

Walk around the gym and hit the machines (which starting strength doesn't use). Instead of squatting as the program calls for you to do, perform some leg isolation exercises. Get creative! As long as you lift some weight and perform different exercises which target the same muscles, you'll be fine. You don't target each and every one but as long as you hit the majority of them, you'll be fine.

The benefit of doing this is that it will get your body used to moving in different ways and will make you stronger in more functional ways. This is over and above the mental benefit of feeling refreshed thanks to the novelty of doing something new. Lastly, it will prevent from falling into a fitness rut where you keep doing the same thing over and over again.

Remember, consistency and a rut are two very different things. The moment you find yourself becoming disillusioned, refresh yourself by doing something else for a week. When you get back to your usual routine, you'll appreciate it more.

Chapter 14 Common Mistakes
People Make

When you are looking to make any significant adjustments in your life. It can take time to discover exactly how to do it in the best ways possible. Many people will make mistakes and have some setbacks as they seek to improve their health through intermittent fasting. Some of these mistakes are minor and can easily be overcome. In contrast, others may be dangerous and could cause serious repercussions if they are not caught in time.

In this chapter, we are going to explore common mistakes that people tend to make when they are on the intermittent fasting diet. We will also explore why these mistakes are made, and how they can be avoided. It is important that you read through this chapter before you commit to the diet itself. That way, you can ensure that you are avoiding any potential mistakes beforehand. This will help you in avoiding unwanted problems and achieving your results with greater success and fewer setbacks.

You should also keep this chapter handy as you embark on your intermittent fasting diet. That way, if you do begin to notice that things are not going as you had hoped, you can easily reflect on this chapter and get the information that you need to adjust your diet and improve your results.

Switching Too Fast

A significant number of people fail to comply with their new diets because they attempt to go too hard too fast. Trying to jump too quickly can result in you feeling too extreme of a departure from your normal. As a result, both psychologically and physically you are put under a significant amount of stress from your new diet. This can lead to you feeling like the diet is not effective and like you are suffering more than you are benefiting from it.

If you are someone who eats regularly and who snacks frequently, switching to the intermittent fasting diet will take time and patience. I cannot stress the importance of your transition period enough.

It is not uncommon to want to jump off the deep end when you are making a lifestyle change. Often, we want to experience great results right away and we are excited about the switch. However, after a few days, it can feel stressful. Because you didn't give your mind and body enough time to adapt to the changes, you ditch your new diet in favor of more comfortable things.

Fasting is something that should always be acclimated to over some time. There is no set period, it needs to be done based on what feels right for you and your body. If you are not properly listening to your body and needs you will end up suffering in major ways. Especially with diets like intermittent fasting, letting yourself adapt to the changes and listening to your body's needs can ensure that you are not neglecting your body in favor of strictly following someone else's guide on what to do.

Choosing the Wrong Plan for Your Lifestyle

It is not uncommon to forget the importance of picking a fasting cycle that actually fits with your lifestyle and then fitting it in. Trying to fast to a cycle that does not fit your lifestyle will ultimately result in you feeling inconvenienced by your diet and struggling to maintain it.

Often, the way we naturally eat is following what we feel fits into our lifestyle in the best way possible. So, if you look at your present diet and notice that there are a lot of convenience meals and they happen all throughout the day, you can conclude two things: you are busy, and you eat when you can. Picking a diet that allows you to eat when you can is important in helping you stick to it. It is also important that you begin searching for healthier convenience options so that you can get the most out of your diet.

Anytime you make a lifestyle change, such as with your diet, you need to consider what your lifestyle actually is. In an ideal world, you may be able to adapt everything to suit your dreamy needs completely. However, in the real world, there are likely many aspects of your lifestyle that are simply not practical to adjust. Picking a diet that suits your lifestyle rather than picking a lifestyle that suits your diet makes far more sense.

Taking the time to actually document what your present eating habits are like before you embark on your intermittent fasting diet is a great way to begin. Focus on what you are already eating and how often and consider diets that will serve your lifestyle. You should also consider your activity levels and how much food you truly need at certain times of the day. For example, if you have a spin class every morning, fasting until noon might not be a good idea as you could end up hungry and exhausted after your class. Choosing the dieting pattern that fits your lifestyle will help you actually maintain your diet so you can continue receiving the great results from it.

Eating Too Much or Not Enough

Focusing on what you are eating and how much you are eating is important. This is one of the biggest reasons why a gradual and intentional transition can be helpful. If you are used to eating throughout the entire day, attempting to eat the same amount in a shorter window can be challenging. You may find yourself feeling stuffed and far too full to actually sustain that amount of eating on a day to day basis. As a result, you may find yourself not eating enough.

Suppose you are new to intermittent fasting and you take the leap too quickly. In that case, it is not unusual to find yourself scarfing down as much food as you possibly can the moment your eating window opens back up. As a result, you find yourself feeling sick, too full, and uncomfortable. Your body also struggles to process and digest that much food after fasting for any given period. This can be even harder on your body if you have been using a more intense fast and then you stuff yourself. If you find yourself doing this, it may be a sign that you have transitioned too quickly and that you need to slow down and back off.

You might also find yourself not eating enough. Attempting to eat the same amount you typically eat in 12-16 hours in just 8-12 hours can be challenging. It may not sound so drastic on paper, but if you are not hungry you may simply not feel like eating. As a result, you may feel compelled to skip meals. This can lead to you not getting enough calories and nutrition in on a daily basis. In the end, you find yourself not eating enough and feeling unsatisfied during your fasting windows.

The best way to combat this is to begin practicing making calorie-dense foods *before* you start intermittent fasting. Learning what recipes you can make and how much each meal needs to have to help you reach your goals is a great way to get yourself ready and show yourself what it truly takes to succeed. Then, begin gradually shortening your eating window and giving yourself the time to work up to eating enough during those eating windows without overeating. In the end, you will find yourself feeling amazing and not feeling unsatisfied or overeating as you maintain your diet.

Your Food Choices are Not Healthy Enough

Even if you are eating according to the keto diet or any other dietary style while intermittently fasting, it is not uncommon to find yourself eating the wrong food choices. Simply knowing what to eat and what to avoid is not enough. You need to spend some time getting to understand what specific vitamins, and minerals you need to thrive. That way, you can eat a diet that is rich in these specific nutrients. Then, you can trust that your body has everything that it needs to thrive on your diet.

Even though intermittent fasting does not technically outline what you should and should not eat, it is not a one-size-fits-all diet that can help you lose weight while eating anything you want. In other words, excessive amounts of junk foods will still hurt you, even if you're eating during the right windows.

You must choose a diet that will help you maintain everything you need to function optimally. Ideally, you should combine intermittent fasting with another diet such as the keto diet, the Mediterranean diet, or any other diet that supports you in eating healthfully. Following the guidelines of these healthier diets ensures that you are incorporating the proper nutrients into your diet so that you can stay healthy.

Eating the right nutrients is essential as it will support your body in healthy hormonal balances and bodily functions. This is how you can keep your organs functioning effectively so that everything works the way it should. As a result, you end up feeling healthier and experiencing greater benefits from your diet. You must focus on this if you want to succeed with your intermittent fasting diet.

You are Not Drinking Enough Fluids

Many people do not realize how much hydration their foods give them on a day to day basis. Food like fruit and vegetables are filled with hydration that supports your body in healthily functions. If you are not eating as many, then you can guarantee that you are not getting as much hydration as you need to be. This means that you need to focus on increasing your hydration levels.

When you are dehydrated you can experience many unwanted symptoms that can make intermittent fasting a challenge. Increased headaches, muscle cramping, and increased hunger are all side effects of dehydration. A great way to combat dehydration is to make sure that you keep water nearby and sip it often. At least once every fifteen minutes to half an hour you should have a good drink of water. This will ensure that you are getting plenty of fresh water into your system.

Other ways to maintain your hydration levels include drinking low-calorie sports drinks, bone broth, tea, and coffee. Essentially, drinking low-calorie drinks throughout the course of the entire day can be extremely helpful in supporting your health. Make sure that you do not exceed your fasting calorie maximum, or you will stop gaining the benefits of fasting. As well, water should always be your first choice above any other drinks to maintain your hydration. However, including some of the others from time to time can support you and keep things interesting so that you can stay hydrated but not bored.

If you begin to experience dehydration symptoms, make sure that you immediately begin increasing the amount of water you are drinking. Dehydration can lead to far more serious side effects beyond headaches and muscle cramps if you are not careful. If you find that you are prone to not drinking enough water daily, consider setting a reminder on your phone that keeps you drinking plenty throughout the day.

The best way to tell that you are staying hydrated enough is to pay attention to how frequently you are peeing. If you are staying in a healthy range of hydration, you should be peeing at least once every single hour. If you aren't, this means that you need to be drinking more water, even if you aren't experiencing any side effects of dehydration. Typically, if you have already begun experiencing side effects then you have waited too long. You want to maintain healthy hydration without waiting for symptoms like headaches and muscle aches to inform you that it is time to start drinking more. This ensures that your body stays happy and healthy and does not cause unnecessary suffering or stress to your body throughout the day.

You are giving up Too Quickly

A lot of people assume that eating the intermittent fasting diet means that they will see the benefits of their eating habits immediately. This is not the case. While intermittent fasting typically offers great results fairly quickly, it does take some time for these results to begin appearing. The exact amount of time depends on many factors. How long it has taken you to transition, what and how you are eating during eating windows, and how much activity you are getting throughout the day contribute to your results.

You might feel compelled to quickly give up if you do not begin noticing your desired results right away, but trust that this is not going to help you. Some people require several weeks before they really begin seeing the benefits of their dieting. This does not mean that it is not working, it simply means that it has taken them some time to find the right balance so that they can gain their desired results and stay healthy.

If you are feeling like throwing in the towel, first take a few minutes to consider what you are doing and how it may be negatively impacting your results. A great way to do this is to try using your food diary once again. For a few days, track how you are eating in accordance with the intermittent fasting diet and what it is doing for you. Get a clear idea of how much you are eating, what you are eating, and when you are eating it. Also, track the amount of physical activity that you are doing on a daily basis.

Through tracking your food intake and exercise levels, you might find that you are not experiencing the results you desire because you are eating too much or not enough in comparison to the amount of energy you are spending each day. Then, you can easily work towards adjusting your diet to find a balance that supports you in getting everything you need and also seeing the results that you desire.

In most cases, intermittent fasting diets are not working because they are not being used right for the individual person. Although the general requirements are somewhat the same, each of us has unique needs based on our lifestyles and our unique makeup. If you are willing to invest time in finding the right balance for yourself then you can guarantee that you can overcome this and experience great results from your fasting.

You are Getting Too Intense or Pushing It

If you are really focused on achieving your desired results, you might feel compelled to push your diet further than what is reasonable for you. For example, attempting to take on too intense of a fasting cycle or trying to do more than your body can reasonably handle. It is not uncommon for people to try and push themselves beyond reasonable measure to achieve their desired results. Unfortunately, this rarely results in them achieving what they actually set out to achieve. It can also have severe consequences.

At the end of the day, listening to your body and paying attention to exactly what it needs is important. You need to be taking care of yourself through proper nutrition and proper exercise levels. You also need to balance these two in a way that serves your body, rather than in a way that leads to you feeling sick and unwell. If you push your body too far, the negative consequences can be severe and long-lasting. In some cases, they may even be life-threatening.

In some cases, pushing your body to a certain extent is necessary. For example, if you are seeking to build more muscle then you want to push yourself to work out enough that your workouts are actually effective. However, if you are pushing yourself to the point that you are beginning to experience negative side effects from your diet, you need to draw back. While certain amounts of side effects are fairly normal early on, experiencing intense side effects, having side effects that don't go away or having them return is not good. You want to work towards maintaining and minimizing your side effects, not constantly living alongside them. After all, what is the point of adjusting your diet and lifestyle to serve your health if you are not actually feeling healthy while you do it?

Make sure that you check in with yourself on a daily basis to see to it that your physical needs are being met. That way, if anything begins to feel excessive or any symptoms begin to increase, you can focus on minimizing or eliminating them right away. Paying close attention to your needs and looking at your goals long-term rather than trying to reach them immediately is the best way to ensure that you reach your health goals without actually compromising your health while attempting to do so. In the end, you will feel much better about doing it this way.

Chapter 15 The Benefits of Fasting For Women Over 50

Studies have shown that intermittent fasting may be extremely useful for postmenopausal women to aid in maintaining their weight. There are quite a few benefits to intermittent fasting for middle-aged women or women that are going through menopause no matter their age.

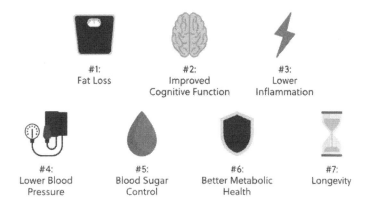

Why for Women Over 50?

Women who approach post-menopause (and sometimes even as early as pre-menopause) tend to start accumulating belly fat. They will start noticing their metabolism get slower. They may also start feeling aches and pains in their joints. Their sleep patterns start to get completely out of routine leaving them feeling exhausted all the time. Then there is the weight gain and also a higher risk of developing chronic diseases like cancer, diabetes, and heart disease that could lead to heart attacks.

There is also the risk of neurodegenerative diseases, stroke, and a constant feeling of fatigue. Intermittent fasting has been known to reset a person's internal balance. This, in turn, boosts their external appearance, energy levels, and cuts down on stress as they control their weight.

Why Should Women Choose the Intermittent Fasting Diet?

Intermittent fasting has become a very popular healthy lifestyle trend, and for good reason. It offers many health benefits as well as improves a person's state of mind and encourages an all-round feeling of well-being.

Benefits of Intermittent Fasting for Women Over 50

When women get to 50 and over, their skin will start to show signs of age. They may find their joints start to ache for no reason, and suddenly belly fat accumulates as if you have just given birth. There are so many creams, diets and exercises on the market to tighten the skin and try to help. The fact is, they may work to a certain point but then the body hits a shelf, and nothing seems to push a person past it. This boils up frustration making women look into the more drastic and very expensive alternatives like surgery. Which in itself poses so many more dangers and risks for women of 50 and over.

A person does not need to go under the knife or starve themselves to reboot their system or change their shape. Intermittent fasting is a much cheaper and less risky way to do this and there is no need to make any drastic eating habit changes either. Well, you may need to make a few adjustments like cutting out junk food and eating healthier. But once again the diet a person follows is their personal choice and depends on how serious they are about becoming healthier.

Some health benefits of intermittent fasting for women over 50 include:

Activating Cellular Repair

Fasting has been known to kick start the body's natural cellular repair function, get rid of mature cells, improve longevity, and improve hormone function. All things that tend to take a battering as people age. This can alleviate joint and muscle aches as well as lower back pain. As the cells are being repaired and damage undone, it helps with the skin's elasticity and health too.

Increase Cognitive Function and Protects the Brain from Damage

Intermittent fasting may increase the levels of a brain hormone known as a brain-derived neurotrophic factor (BDNF). It may equally guard the brain against damage like a stroke or Alzheimer's disease as it promotes new nerve cell growth. It also increases cognitive function and could effectively defend a person against other neurodegenerative diseases as well.

Weight Loss

When people have belly fat, it can cause many health problems that are associated with various diseases as it indicates a person has visceral fat. Visceral fat is fat that goes deep into the abdominal surrounding the organs. Belly fat is terribly hard to lose, especially for an aging woman. Intermittent fasting has been known to help reduce not only weight but inches of over five percent of body fat in around twenty-two to twenty-five weeks (Barna, 2019).

Alleviates Oxidative Stress and Inflammation

Oxidative stress is when the body has an imbalance of antioxidants as well as free radicals. This imbalance can cause both tissue and cell damage in overweight as well as aging people. It can also lead to various chronic illnesses like cancer, heart disease, diabetes, and also has an impact on the signs of aging. Oxidative stress can trigger the inflammation that causes these diseases.

Intermittent fasting can provide your system with a reboot, helping to alleviate oxidative stress and inflammation in a middle-aged woman. It also significantly reduces the risk of oxidative stress and inflammation for those overweight or obese.

Slow Down the Aging Process

As intermittent fasting gives both the metabolism and cellular repair a reboot it offers the potential to slow down aging. It may even prolong a person's lifespan by quite a few years especially if following a nutritious diet and exercise regime alongside intermittent fasting.

Chapter 16 Recipes

1. Blueberries Breakfast Bowl

Preparation time 35 minutes

Cooking time: 0 minutes

Servings: 1

Ingredients:

1-tsp chia seeds

1-cup almond milk

¼-cup fresh blueberries or fresh fruits

1-pack sweetener for taste

Directions:

Mix the chia seeds with almond milk. Stir periodically.

Place in the fridge to cool for 30 minutes, and then serve with fresh fruit. Enjoy!

Nutrition:

Calories: 202

Fat: 16.8g

Protein: 10.2g

Total Carbohydrates: 9.8g

Dietary Fiber: 5.8g

Net Carbohydrates: 2.6g

2. Feta-Filled Tomato-Topped Oldie Omelet

Preparation time 5 minutes

Cooking time: 6 minutes

Servings: 1

Ingredients:

1-tbsp coconut oil

2-pcs eggs

1½-tbsp milk

A dash of salt and pepper

¼-cup tomatoes, sliced into cubes

2-tbsp feta cheese, crumbled

Directions:

Beat the eggs with the pepper, salt, milk, and the remaining spices.

Pour the mixture into a heated pan with coconut oil.

Stir in the tomatoes and cheese. Cook for 6 minutes or until the cheese melts.

Nutrition:

Calories: 335

Fat: 28.4g

Protein: 16.2g

Total Carbohydrates: 4.5g

Dietary Fiber: 0.8g

Net Carbohydrates: 3.7g

3. Carrot Breakfast Salad

Preparation time: 5 minutes

Cooking time: 4 hours

Servings: 4

Ingredients:

2 tablespoons olive oil

2 pounds baby carrots, peeled and halved

3 garlic cloves, minced

2 yellow onions, chopped

½ cup vegetable stock

1/3 cup tomatoes, crushed

A pinch of salt and black pepper

Directions:

In your slow cooker, combine all the ingredients, cover and cook on high for 4 hours.

Divide into bowls and serve for breakfast.

Nutrition:

Calories: 437 kcal

Protein: 2.39 g

Fat: 39.14 g

Carbohydrates: 23.28 g

4. Paprika Lamb Chops

Preparation time 10 minutes

Cooking time: 15 minutes

Servings: 4

 Ingredients:

2 lamb racks, cut into chops

Salt and pepper to taste

3 tablespoons paprika

¾ cup cumin powder

1 teaspoon chili powder

Directions:

Take a bowl and add paprika, cumin, chili, salt, pepper, and stir.

Add lamb chops and rub the mixture

Heat grill over medium-temperature and add lamb chops, cook for 5 minutes

Flip and cook for 5 minutes more, flip again.

Cook for 2 minutes, flip and cook for 2 minutes more

Serve and enjoy!

Nutrition:

Calories: 200

Fat: 5g

Carbohydrates: 4g

Protein: 8g

5. Delicious Tur key Wrap

Preparation time 10 minutes

Cooking time: 10 minutes

Servings: 6

Ingredients:1 and a ¼ pounds of ground turkey, lean - 4 green onions, minced

1 tablespoon of olive oil - 1 garlic clove, minced

2 teaspoon of chili paste

8-ounce water chestnut, diced

3 tablespoon of hoisin sauce

2 tablespoon of coconut aminos

1 tablespoon of rice vinegar

12 butter lettuce leaves

1/8 teaspoon of salt

Directions:

Take a pan and place it over medium heat, add turkey and garlic to the pan

Heat for 6 minutes until cooked

Take a bowl and transfer turkey to the bowl

Add onions and water chestnuts

Stir in hoisin sauce, coconut aminos, vinegar, and chili paste

Toss well and transfer the mix to lettuce leaves

Serve and enjoy!

Nutrition: Calories: 162 Fat: 4g Net Carbohydrates: 7g Protein: 23g

6. Bacon and Chicken Garlic Wrap

Preparation time 15 minutes

Cooking time: 10 minutes

Servings: 4

 Ingredients:

1 chicken fillet, cut into small cubes

8-9 thin slices bacon, cut to fit cubes

6 garlic cloves, minced

Directions:

Preheat your oven to 400 degrees F

Line a baking tray with aluminum foil

Add minced garlic to a bowl and rub each chicken piece with it

Wrap bacon piece around each garlic chicken bite

Secure with toothpick

Transfer bites to the baking sheet, keeping a little bit of space between them

Bake for about 15-20 minutes until crispy

Serve and enjoy!

Nutrition:

Calories: 260

Fat: 19g

Carbohydrates: 5g

Protein: 22g Dinner Recipes

7. Coated Cauliflower Head

Preparation time: 10 minutes

Cooking time: 40 minutes

Servings: 6

Ingredients: 2-pound cauliflower head

3 tablespoons olive oil

1 tablespoon butter, softened

1 teaspoon ground coriander

1 teaspoon salt

1 egg, whisked

1 teaspoon dried cilantro

1 teaspoon dried oregano

1 teaspoon tahini paste

Directions:

Trim cauliflower head if needed.

Preheat oven to 350F.

In the mixing bowl, mix up together olive oil, softened butter, ground coriander, salt, whisked egg, dried cilantro, dried oregano, and tahini paste.

Then brush the cauliflower head with this mixture generously and transfer in the tray.

Bake the cauliflower head for 40 minutes.

Brush it with the remaining oil mixture every 10 minutes.

Nutrition: Calories: 136 kcal Protein: 4.43 g Fat: 10.71 g

Carbohydrates: 7.8 g

8. Cauliflower Crust Pizza

Preparation time: 20 minutes

Cooking time: 42 minutes

Servings: 2

Allergens: egg, dairy

Ingredients: For Crust: - 1 small head cauliflower, cut into florets - 2 large organic eggs, beaten lightly

½ teaspoon dried oregano - ½ teaspoon garlic powder - Ground black pepper, as required

For Topping: - ½ cup sugar-free pizza sauce - ¾ cup mozzarella cheese, shredded

¼ cup black olives, pitted and sliced - 2 tablespoons Parmesan cheese, grated

Directions:

Preheat your oven to 4000 F (2000 C). Line a baking sheet with a lightly greased parchment paper. Add the cauliflower in a food processor and pulse until rice like texture is achieved. In a bowl, add the cauliflower rice, eggs, oregano, garlic powder, and black pepper and mix until well combined. Place the cauliflower the mixture in the center of the prepared baking sheet and with a spatula, press into a 13-inch thin circle. Bake for 40 minutes or until golden-brown. Remove the baking sheet from the oven. Now, set the oven to broiler on high. Place the tomato sauce on top of the pizza crust and with a spatula, spread evenly and sprinkle with olives, followed by the cheeses. Broil for about 1-2 minutes or until the cheese is bubbly and browned. Remove from oven and with a pizza cutter, cut the pizza into equal sized triangles. Serve hot.

Nutrition:

Calories: 119 Fat: 6.6g Sat Fat: 1.8g

Cholesterol: 98mg Sodium: 297mg Carbohydrates: 8.6g

Fiber: 3.4g Sugar: 3.7g Protein: 8.3g

9. Cabbage Casserole

Preparation time: 15 minutes

Cooking time: 30 minutes

Servings: 2

Allergens: dairy

Ingredients: ½ head cabbage - 2 scallions, chopped - 4 tablespoons unsalted butter

2 ounces cream cheese, softened - ¼ cup Parmesan cheese, grated

¼ cup fresh cream - ½ teaspoon Dijon mustard - 2 tablespoons fresh parsley, chopped

Salt and ground black pepper, as required

Directions

Preheat your oven to 3500 F (1800 C).

Cut cabbage head into half, lengthwise. Then cut into 4 equal sized wedges.

In a pan of boiling water, add cabbage wedges and cook, covered for about 5 minutes.

Drain well and arrange cabbage wedges into a small baking dish.

In a small pan, melt butter and sauté onions for about 5 minutes.

Add the remaining ingredients and stir to combine.

Remove from the heat and immediately, place the cheese mixture over cabbage wedges evenly.

Bake for about 20 mins.

Remove from the oven and let it cool for about 5 minutes before serving.

Cut into 3 equal sized portions and serve.

Nutrition Calories: 273 Fat: 24.8g Sat Fat: 15.4g

Cholesterol: 71mg Sodium: 313mg Carbohydrates: 9g Fiber: 3.4g Sugar: 4.5g Protein: 6.2g

10. Salmon with Salsa

Preparation time: 15 minutes

Cooking time: 8 minutes

Servings: 2

Allergens: dairy

Ingredients: For Salsa: - 1 small tomato, chopped

2 tablespoons red onion, chopped finely - ¼ cup fresh cilantro, chopped finely

1 tablespoon jalapeño pepper, seeded and minced finely - 1 garlic clove, minced finely

Salt and ground black pepper, as required - For Salmon: - 4 (5-ounce) (1-inch thick) salmon fillets

3 tablespoons butter - 1 tablespoon fresh rosemary leaves, chopped - 1 tablespoon fresh lemon juice

Directions

For salsa: Add all ingredients in a bowl and gently, stir to combine. With a plastic wrap, cover the bowl and refrigerate before serving. For salmon: season each salmon fillet with salt and black pepper generously. In a large skillet, melt butter over medium-high. Place the salmon fillets, skins side up and cook for about 4 minutes. Carefully change the side of each salmon fillet and cook for about 4 minutes more. Stir in the rosemary and lemon juice and remove from the heat. Divide the salsa onto serving plates evenly. To each plate with 1 salmon fillet and serve.

Nutrition:

Calories: 481 Fat: 37.2g Sat Fat: 10.9g

Cholesterol: 85mg Sodium: 172mg Carbohydrates: 11g

Fiber: 7.6g Sugar: 1.5g Protein: 29.9g

11. Artichoke Petals Bites

Preparation time: 10 minutes

Cooking time: 10 minutes

Servings: 8

Ingredients:

8 oz artichoke petals, boiled, drained, without salt

½ cup almond flour

4 oz Parmesan, grated

2 tablespoons almond butter, melted

Directions:

In the mixing bowl, mix up together almond flour and grated Parmesan.

Preheat the oven to 355F.

Dip the artichoke petals in the almond butter and then coat in the almond flour mixture.

Could you place them in the tray?

Transfer the tray in the preheated oven and cook the petals for 10 minutes.

Chill the cooked petal bites little before serving.

Nutrition:

Calories: 93 kcal

Protein: 6.54 g

Fat: 3.72 g

Carbohydrates: 9.08 g

12. Stuffed Beef Loin in Sticky Sauce

Preparation time: 15 minutes

Cooking time: 6 minutes

Servings: 4

Ingredients: 1 tablespoon Erythritol - 1 tablespoon lemon juice - 4 tablespoons water

1 tablespoon butter - ½ teaspoon tomato sauce - ¼ teaspoon dried rosemary

9 oz beef loin - 3 oz celery root, grated - 3 oz bacon, sliced - 1 tablespoon walnuts, chopped

¾ teaspoon garlic, diced 2 teaspoons butter - 1 tablespoon olive oil - 1 teaspoon salt - ½ cup of water

Directions:

Cut the beef loin into the layer and spread it with the dried rosemary, butter, and salt. Then place over the beef loin: grated celery root, sliced bacon, walnuts, and diced garlic. Roll the beef loin and brush it with olive oil. Secure the meat with the help of the toothpicks. Please place it in the tray and add a ½ cup of water. Cook the meat in the preheated to 365F oven for 40 minutes. Meanwhile, make the sticky sauce: mix up together Erythritol, lemon juice, 4 tablespoons of water, and butter. Preheat the mixture until it starts to boil. Then add tomato sauce and whisk it well. Bring the sauce to boil and remove from the heat. When the beef loin is cooked, please remove it from the oven and brush with the cooked sticky sauce very generously. Slice the beef roll and sprinkle with the remaining sauce.

Nutrition:

Calories: 321 kcal

Protein: 18.35 g

Fat: 26.68 g

Carbohydrates: 2.75 g

13. Eggplant Fries

Preparation time 10 minutes

Cooking time: 15 minutes

Servings: 8

Ingredients:

2 eggs

2 cups almond flour

2 tablespoons coconut oil, spray

2 eggplant, peeled and cut thinly

Salt and pepper

Directions:

Preheat your oven to 400 degrees Fahrenheit

Take a bowl and mix with salt and black pepper in it

Take another bowl and beat eggs until frothy

Dip the eggplant pieces into eggs

Then coat them with flour mixture

Add another layer of flour and egg

Then, take a baking sheet and grease with coconut oil on top

Bake for about 15 minutes

Serve and enjoy!

Nutrition

Calories: 212 Fat: 15.8g Carbohydrates: 12.1g Protein: 8.6g

14. Parmesan Crisps

Preparation time 5 minutes

Cooking time: 25 minutes

Servings: 8

Ingredients:

1 teaspoon butter

8 ounces parmesan cheese, full fat and shredded

Directions:

Preheat your oven to 400 degrees F

Put parchment paper on a baking sheet and grease with butter

Spoon parmesan into 8 mounds, spreading them apart evenly

Flatten them

Bake for 5 minutes until browned

Let them cool

Serve and enjoy!

Nutrition:

Calories: 133

Fat: 11g

Carbohydrates: 1g

Protein: 11g

15. Roasted Broccoli

Preparation time 5 minutes

Cooking time: 20 minutes

Servings: 4

 Ingredients:

4 cups broccoli florets

1 tablespoon olive oil

Salt and pepper to taste

Directions:

Preheat your oven to 400 degrees F

Add broccoli in a zip bag alongside oil and shake until coated

Add seasoning and shake again

Spread broccoli out on the baking sheet, bake for 20 minutes

Let it cool and serve

Enjoy!

Nutrition:

Calories: 62

Fat: 4g

Carbohydrates: 4g

Protein: 4g

Conclusion

Intermittent fasting can be very challenging at first but if you can get over the few times and stick to it, it is immensely rewarding.

Don't give up if you feel that the fasting plan you have chosen is too much for you. Ask your medical advisor to help you either modify your current plan or try another one. Not everyone is suited to each plan. You may find you need to try one or two before you are comfortable.

You don't have to dive right into adjusting your eating habits as well as try intermittent fasting all at once either. Start off fasting, eating normally but cutting down and gradually make food choice changes as you become more comfortable with fasting.

The trick is to find your balance, one step at a time if you must, as long as you are working to your end goal. How long it takes to get you there is entirely up to you. Don't think you have to rush headlong into it. Set achievable realistic goals that you feel one hundred percent comfortable with, otherwise your intermittent fasting diet is not going to work.

This is a lifestyle change, not a fad diet that you try for a few days or weeks and then forget because it became mundane or too challenging. This is a diet and lifestyle you need to commit to that will not only help you lose weight but be beneficial for your health. There is nothing wrong with easing into it; it is not a race and you have to remember you are doing this for you!

Well done on your decision to make a choice to try the intermittent fasting and all the very best. You can do this — you have got this!

Manufactured by Amazon.ca
Bolton, ON